THE FRAGMENTED SELF, RECOGNITION, AND THE EDGE OF DESIRE

This book explores the most unstable facets of psychic life and how these can be understood and engaged in the psychoanalytic consulting room.

Psychic life is sustained by its very instabilities—by fragmentation, paradox, and the defenses that make survival possible. In dialogue with both psychoanalytic and philosophical traditions, Anderson shows how analysis becomes an aesthetic practice of presence, one that sustains the paradoxes necessary for psychic vitality. Reframing foundational psychoanalytic concepts such as the false self, regression, and symbolization, this book develops a clinical lens attuned to ambiguity, embodiment, and survival. Drawing from relational and post-structuralist traditions, it weaves vivid clinical vignettes with theoretical inquiry to explore how the psyche organizes itself around absence, symbolic rupture, and ethical refusal.

With a distinctive perspective on subjectivity, this book offers an aesthetic and ethical framework for psychoanalysis—one that sustains engagement with paradox, dissociation, and symbolic survival over premature resolution. It is essential reading for psychoanalysts, psychotherapists, and scholars of psychoanalytic thought.

Todd Anderson, PhD, PsyD, is a psychoanalyst practicing in New York City. His work explores how dissociation and desire shape psychic survival, bringing together insights from object relations, relational psychoanalysis, and contemporary philosophy.

Psychoanalysis in a New Key
Donnel Stern
Series Editor

When music is played in a new key, the melody does not change, but the notes that make up the composition do: change in the context of continuity, continuity that perseveres through change. Psychoanalysis in a New Key publishes books that share the aims psychoanalysts have always had, but that approach them differently. The books in the series are not expected to advance any particular theoretical agenda, although to this date most have been written by analysts from the Interpersonal and Relational orientations.

The most important contribution of a psychoanalytic book is the communication of something that nudges the reader's grasp of clinical theory and practice in an unexpected direction. Psychoanalysis in a New Key creates a deliberate focus on innovative and unsettling clinical thinking. Because that kind of thinking is encouraged by exploration of the sometimes surprising contributions to psychoanalysis of ideas and findings from other fields, Psychoanalysis in a New Key particularly encourages interdisciplinary studies. Books in the series have married psychoanalysis with dissociation, trauma theory, sociology, and criminology. The series is open to the consideration of studies examining the relationship between psychoanalysis and any other field—for instance, biology, literary and art criticism, philosophy, systems theory, anthropology, and political theory.

But innovation also takes place within the boundaries of psychoanalysis, and Psychoanalysis in a New Key therefore also presents work that reformulates thought and practice without leaving the precincts of the field. Books in the series focus, for example, on the significance of personal values in psychoanalytic practice, on the complex interrelationship between the analyst's clinical work and personal life, on the consequences for the clinical situation when patient and analyst are from different cultures, and on the need for psychoanalysts to accept the degree to which they knowingly satisfy their own wishes during treatment hours, often to the patient's detriment.

A full list of all titles in this series is available at: https://www.routledge.com/Psychoanalysis-in-a-New-Key-Book-Series/book-series/LEAPNKBS

"Brilliant, compelling, and thought-provoking."

Christopher Bollas, PhD, *author of* The Shadow of the Object *and* Being a Character

"I find *Unstable Objects* to be a book that manages to describe the phenomena constituting the analytic experience in an unusually delicate and intelligent way. This is a rare event in the analytic world. It is a pleasure to read."

Thomas Ogden, MD, *author of* What Alive Means *and* Coming to Life in the Consulting Room

"Taking the centrality of conflict, contradiction, and paradox in mental life as his subject of investigation, Todd Anderson offers us a discourse of astonishing range and depth. His approach integrates the perspectives of classical psychoanalysis, contemporary intersubjectivity, and modern Continental philosophy. The labyrinthine and near-mesmerizing syncretism that marks his voice yields proposals that are thoughtful, convincing, and humane. Paradox is thus revealed to be integral, inevitable, and, if held by unhurried attention, deeply instructive as well. This is a truly meaningful addition to our current psychoanalytic literature!"

Salman Akhtar, MD, DLFAPA, *emeritus professor of Psychiatry, Jefferson Medical College; training and supervising analyst, Psychoanalytic Center of Philadelphia*

"When you begin to read Todd Anderson's two-volume *Unstable Objects*, one of the more remarkable debut efforts to appear in our psychoanalytic literature, you will immediately feel, as I did when I first encountered this work, that you are in the hands of a master, someone who thinks with rare depth and grace, and whose writing is—what should I say?—simply marvelous. It's not just that Anderson writes beautifully and with great expressiveness. He does. But he also writes in a way that makes it virtually effortless to read him, even when he addresses complex matters. As lovely as it is, the writing is always transparent to the subject matter. Anderson's modesty, simplicity, and quiet confidence allow him to approach profound psychoanalytic questions with great thoughtfulness. In the process, he adds to our appreciation of the work of analytic writers, and others, who have preceded him. Over and over again, the writing demands quotation. You will find yourself trying to get people, especially people who know psychoanalysis, to listen to the many passages that say something in words that, once read, are irreplaceable. These books are special. They constitute a kind of manifesto, a statement of the nature of psychoanalysis from Anderson's relational point of view. Do yourself a favor: Read them."

Donnel B. Stern, PhD, *William Alanson White Institute; NYU Postdoctoral Program*

"This book doesn't simply present ideas; it evokes states of mind. The writing form itself becomes part of the witnessing process—recursive, atmospheric, and affectively alive. Todd Anderson carries forward a lineage of symbolic containment that allows what is fragile, unformulated, and reverent to be held without being prematurely resolved. This is a work of psychoanalysis as living process."

Michael Eigen, PhD, *author of* The Psychoanalytic Mystic *and* The Sensitive Self

"Todd Anderson's new book makes me want to go back and rewrite everything I've ever published—not out of regret, but because of how deeply he integrates the loose ends of so many theorists we share and love. His work is a tour de force: richly lived in, deliberately untidy, and fiercely humane. Anderson writes not to our 'churches of reason,' but from within the clinical hour itself. He invites us to dwell in contradiction—not to interpret or resolve, but to inhabit. This is psychoanalysis at its most human: not aiming to fix, but to move, to dwell, to return home."

Philip Ringstrom, PhD, *author of* A Relational Psychoanalytic Approach to Couples Psychotherapy

"Each practitioner must make psychoanalysis in their own idiom, personalizing theory to hold us as we reach for authenticity in clinical engagement. Todd Anderson offers original ways to understand the shapes and contours of the relationships we encounter as we try to make sense of the therapy that helps both us and our analysands."

Susie Orbach, PhD, *author of* Fat Is a Feminist Issue *and featured in* Expanding Psychoanalysis: The Contributions of Susie Orbach (*edited by Brett Kahr*)

"A remarkable new voice has been added to the canon of contemporary psychoanalytic writing. With startling originality, Todd Anderson deconstructs the earliest expressions of subjectivity and the ways in which they can go awry. He finds ways to frame and elaborate theoretical material that is at once familiar yet his fresh and compelling insights encourage clinicians to look further. These volumes will become an essential addition to our professional libraries."

Ghislaine Boulanger, PhD, *author of* Wounded by Reality: Understanding *and* Treating Adult Onset Trauma

The Fragmented Self, Recognition, and the Edge of Desire

Foundations of the Psychoanalysis of Unstable Objects

Todd Anderson

Routledge
Taylor & Francis Group
LONDON AND NEW YORK

Designed cover image: Getty Images

First published 2026
by Routledge
4 Park Square, Milton Park, Abingdon, Oxon OX14 4RN

and by Routledge
605 Third Avenue, New York, NY 10158

Routledge is an imprint of the Taylor & Francis Group, an informa business

British Library Cataloguing-in-Publication Data
A catalogue record for this book is available from the British Library

ISBN: 9781041201489 (hbk)
ISBN: 9781041171485 (pbk)
ISBN: 9781003715283 (ebk)

DOI: 10.4324/9781003715283

Typeset in Optima
by codeMantra

For Nancy McWilliams—for seeing something I hadn't yet lived into, and for coaxing it forth with warmth, faith, and fierce encouragement.

For Donnel Stern—for your generous enthusiasm and quiet conviction, and for meeting me on the path as a fellow traveler in the field of experience.

To you both—thank you for taking my thinking seriously, before I was certain it deserved to be.

Contents

Overture—The Call Before Being

Why Think?

Every critique already constructs, every construction already critiques—yet my work takes up where Foucault's genealogies leave off, emphasizing the constructive task. Construction is more difficult, for it requires submission to the imperfections of language, symbolization, and communication itself. Nothing that can be spoken or known will ever be fully true. Yet to say nothing is to abandon the possibility of resonance—the chance that words, however partial, might evoke truth in another.

Critique and construction are never opposites. To construct is already to exclude, to delimit, to undo. To deconstruct is already to build, to open, to make possible. My work seeks to explore this entanglement: how every construction deconstructs and how every deconstruction necessarily constructs. In this reciprocal knot, psychoanalysis finds its most fertile ground.

Psychoanalysis has too often been confined to epistemology—as a science of unconscious knowledge—or to ontology—as a discourse on being, presence, and psychic structure. I envision it otherwise: in the same pre-ontological register Levinas explores—where the face of the Other calls us into responsibility before we can know or even be. Ferenczi, Laplanche, and Loewald each remind us, in their different ways, that analytic life is organized not around what we know or who we are, but around the summons, the enigmatic address, the unformulated demand that comes before subjectivity itself.

In this horizon, interpretation does not secure truth or consolidate being; it answers. Always inadequately, but always necessarily. Here Donna Orange's Levinasian ethic of responsibility is indispensable: psychoanalysis is not a project of epistemic mastery, but an infinite responsibility to and for the Other, borne in the fragile act of speech itself. And as Thomas Ogden shows, analytic thought lives in paradox: every interpretation is both form and dissolution, every symbol both construction and deconstruction. To think is to enact this doubleness, to inhabit the entanglement it describes.

Why think? Because thought itself is a mode of response. To think, to analyze, to construct, is to answer the call that comes before being. To take responsibility for what we share—our imperfect knowings and unknowings—so that, through their very incompleteness, they may evoke meaning and sustain the fragile work of living and knowing with others. To think is to answer the call before being—never completely, never finally, but always as an act of responsibility.

Foreword to Todd Anderson's *Unstable Objects*

It is my great honor and pleasure to write a foreword to this two-volume work. I originally met Todd Anderson when he contacted me in the spring of 2024 to ask, rather shyly, if I could consult with him regularly on his cases. We had had no prior connection; he explained his reaching out to me in terms of his sense that we might work well together on deepening his understanding of patients. We agreed to consult once or twice a month by phone. Our early meetings involved both clinical consultations and efforts on my part to help him contain his exasperation as he faced various infantilizing professional hassles, including some mundane and pedantic bureaucratic hoops he was jumping through at the time. I noticed that he had a fine intuition and an unusual degree of intelligence and intellectual creativity.

When we talked about cases, Todd would describe his patients with exquisitely evocative, spontaneous metaphors that captured their uniqueness. He was consistently collaborative and never defensive. He reacted to my thoughts about his clients with an interest that was both open-minded and open-hearted. As we worked on clinical and professional issues, it became clear that Todd is a person for whom psychoanalysis has been more than a discipline that enables one to conceptualize personality dynamics and the psychotherapy process. For him, the analytic tradition, which he aptly calls "a strange hybrid genre: part philosophy, part science, part testimony, part literature," has been a lifeline and a calling. Todd is the rare individual whose search for meaning is uncontaminated by petty ambitions and competitions; it encompasses all aspects of his personal and vocational being. It often felt to me as if his central mission was simply to name what felt true. That much I had begun to understand about him when I first learned that he also likes to write.

A few months ago, toward the end of a consultation session, Todd mentioned rather casually that he had written a few essays about psychoanalytic topics. I volunteered to look at anything he had written and think with him about whether it might be publishable, and if so, where to send it. He seemed pleased, and a bit surprised, and emailed me a couple of attachments, essays that have turned into chapters in this two-volume contribution. When I sat down to read what he had written, I was stunned. The mind of this modest, unassuming guy was awash in brilliant, original insights. He has the extraordinary ability of only a very few analysts—Thomas Ogden, Michael Eigen, and Donnel Stern come to mind, thinkers with whom he recognizes a shared sensibility—to talk about what is in one way obvious and in another way invisible. He can hold multiple theoretical orientations in simultaneous, layered, even holographic thinking, drawing from each without being confined by any. And the man can write.

The effect of Todd's gorgeous prose was to put me into a trancelike state that I have entered only a few times when reading professional literature. That response more often happens when I am in the presence of the spiritual, the ineffable, and the profound; it is how I experience music and poetry but not usually psychoanalytic theory. As readers can see from the book jacket endorsements, I am not alone in that reaction. Todd has and is, as Ghislaine Boulanger notes, a remarkable new voice. I am going to enjoy his bursting on the analytic scene after all his quiet, private meditations on the great human questions with which our discipline at its best is always grappling. Let me introduce you to Todd's singular idiom.

This is a voice that is both humble and confident, matter-of-fact and lyrical, soothing and startling. It is provocative without the aggression that provocation usually includes. It reverberates. The harsh conditions of Todd's upbringing in rural Kentucky, combined with the loneliness inherent in an intelligence that is about four standard deviations above the mean, have situated him again and again at the margins, a location that gives him perspective that those in the center cannot easily attain. In a metaphor that he would find too stale for his own writing, Todd finds himself in these books trying to describe water to fish.

Todd's way of thinking is intrinsically holistic. On the Rorschach, he would probably give whole-card responses to every inkblot. The terrain of his mental landscape is constantly lit up by images and metaphors. They arise in his consciousness as highly condensed messages from his lived experience. Then, like a jazz musician with a melodic theme, he riffs. He lets himself be taken over by his mental wanderings, reflects on them with the help of his impressive erudition until he feels he understands something of value, and then, as when one's water breaks at the end of a pregnancy, the words pour out of him. After a gestation period of several years, Todd wrote this two-volume manuscript in a few weeks.

This book exemplifies what it tries to depict. It is recursive. It embraces paradox. It will expand your thinking in welcome ways, introduce you to ideas you thought you understood but had not considered in their full implications, and provide the "Aha!" experience that the analytic community once idealized as the emotional consequence of an elegant interpretation. The sheer vitality in Todd's excursions will energize your mind, and you will enjoy the writing in the same way you appreciate a fine novel or short story. It is a privilege to introduce to my psychoanalytic colleagues this evocative work, a contribution that I believe will help shape the next chapter of our field.

Nancy McWilliams
Visiting Professor Emerita, Rutgers
Graduate School of Applied &
Professional Psychology
August 31, 2025

Opening Notes

On Form

This book draws on what I call the *Lineage of Remainder* in psychoanalysis: a current of voices that remind us of what cannot be fully integrated or domesticated. Christopher Bollas has spoken of the unthought known, Michael Eigen of storms of affect, Thomas Ogden of an analytic third that exceeds any one subjectivity, and Donnel Stern of unformulated experience and dissociation. Each points toward the residue, the excess, the paradox that resists closure. This book continues in that lineage, suggesting that *remainder* is not a flaw in our theories but the vital condition of psychic life.

This book is written with the utmost precision. It tracks fragmentation, dissociation, affective charge, and the presence of the unknown with unwavering attention. That precision requires a prose style that is nonlinear, formally exacting, and at times unconventional.

The form, too, speaks: the medium is part of the message.

Like Cage's *4'33"*, Duchamp's *Fountain*, or Stravinsky's *Rite of Spring*, this work asks you to relinquish the usual stance of interpretive presumption. It repositions the reader. It alters the frame.

I have written from within these topics, relinquishing the more usual stance of writing about them.

Demands for clarity often function to silence what disturbs. As Glissant reminds us, the call for transparency is often a colonial imposition—a refusal of the right to opacity. Foucault teaches that regimes of intelligibility are also regimes of power—shaping what can be said, seen, or known. And as Derrida insists, meaning always slips—every effort to stabilize it is already haunted by what it excludes. Intelligibility, then, is never neutral; it is both a practice of power and a defense against what resists containment.

As Audre Lorde taught, the master's tools will never dismantle the master's house.

The myth of standard form and cogent style is not a path to truth, but a technique of containment.

This book stays with the tension of what resists premature coherence.

At the heart of this project is what I would describe as structural humility—the recognition that every interpretation is partial, every theoretical frame a form of containment rather than revelation. Psychoanalytic concepts are indispensable, but they are not final. The psyche will always exceed them.

I have refrained from the epistemological violence of privileging clarity or legibility over truth and presence.

Hans Loewald reminds us that symbolization is not description, but transformation. This book participates in that act. It does not translate the psyche. It transmits it.

I have privileged cultivating an experience of the terrain over delivering a clean, internally coherent, and ultimately generic map.

The writing embodies the Levinasian ethic of the infinite—without totalizing. It offers no final understanding, only a sustained proximity.

A Recursive Ethic

The form of these texts follows a Levinasian ethic of recursion. Rather than advancing through linear argument, accumulating evidence, or arriving at closure, the writing turns back on itself—circling, revisiting, and re-marking what came before. This recursive movement enacts what Emmanuel Levinas called the infinite responsibility to the face of the other: an ethical demand that precedes comprehension and resists completion. The writing remains asymmetrically responsive to what cannot be fully known, integrating rupture, contradiction, and unformulated experience as essential. It bends toward what exceeds understanding—form as ethical exposure, language as an act of sustained, non-mastering presence. In this way, the rhythm of the text mirrors the clinical situation itself, where understanding emerges not through deduction but through shared atmosphere, affective resonance, and the return of what has not yet been symbolized.

This writing engages each concept not to contain or resolve it, but to open a field of symbolic resonance. Its form reflects an aesthetic epistemology, where truth is approached as a lived, relational process—held in texture, pacing, image, and tone. Each chapter structures itself as a mode of listening, shaped by the atmosphere of what cannot be directly spoken. Concepts are carried as intensities rather than explained as conclusions. This sensibility draws from psychoanalytic traditions that privilege emergence over interpretation and remain faithful to what resists formulation. The text itself becomes a space of attunement.

For some readers, especially those more accustomed to linear argument, the recursive structure may evoke disorientation, pause, or repetition. These qualities are not ornamental but deliberate: they echo the experience of unconscious life and the process of analytic work. The form draws on writers within psychoanalysis—including Bion, Ogden, Eigen, and Bollas—who transmit psychic truth through mood, pattern, atmosphere, and symbolic layering. Each return marks a shift; each hesitation allows something unsymbolized to enter. The writing offers not a path to conclusion, but an invitation to dwell in the presence of what stirs, fragments, or remains just beyond reach. In that space, recognition becomes a felt event, not a finished product.

On Symbolic Form

This book unfolds within a symbolic form where language holds more than it says. Its architecture is recursive, affective, and veiled—not to obscure meaning, but to allow it to arrive slowly, elliptically, and in fragments. Here, form is not decoration. It is a symbolic architecture—a topology of thought that permits certain truths to become speakable without being flattened.

There is a quiet lineage of psychoanalytic thinkers who have worked in this form, the *Lineage of Remainder*. Hans Loewald wrote with a soft, recursive gravity, composing a poetics of symbolic containment where psyche and world co-emerge.[1] Christopher Bollas shaped atmospheres of associative drift that preserved the evocative unknown.[2] Michael Eigen offered trembling fragments that held affect without resolution.[3] Jean Laplanche structured theory around the enigmatic, insisting on the radical latency of meaning.[4] André Green mapped the syntax of absence, showing how psychic life organizes around the ungraspable.[5]

These writers did not merely describe experience—they created forms that could contain it. Their work gave shape to meaning without dislocating it from the body, from affect, or from the unconscious. What they built—implicitly or explicitly—was a recursive epistemology, in which the form itself becomes an act of witnessing.

This book continues that inheritance. Its recursive grammar was not chosen for aesthetic effect; it arose out of necessity. To translate these ideas into linear exposition would be to disfigure them. The form protects what clarity would dissolve. It offers a delayed arrival for truths that cannot be directly held.

Here, delay, veiling, and symbolic resonance are not literary devices. They are ethical responses to the unspeakable. They allow psychic realities to unfold on their own terms, in their own tempo, without being forced into coherence.

For some readers, this will feel unfamiliar. But for others—for those who have long lived in nonlinear space, who recognize that knowing sometimes requires a detour—this form will not need justification. It will feel like home.

The glow you notice isn't free-floating—it's light diffused through fog. The atmosphere is real, but it needs a medium to live in.

Notes

1 Loewald, H. W. (1980). *Psychoanalysis and the future*. International Universities Press.
2 Bollas, C. (1987). *The shadow of the object: Psychoanalysis of the unthought known*. Columbia University Press.
3 Eigen, M. (2004). *The sensitive self.* Wesleyan University Press.
4 Laplanche, J. (1999). *Essays on otherness* (J. Fletcher, Trans.). Routledge.
5 Green, A. (1999). *The work of the negative* (A. Weller, Trans.). Free Association Books.

Acknowledgments

This book has emerged through a long field of influence, reading, and relational presence. Its thinking is shaped as much by the silences I've sat with as by the voices I've studied. I want to thank a few of those who have marked the work, held its formation, or witnessed its becoming.

To Nancy McWilliams, for your generosity, steadiness, and capacity to see what is not yet formed. Your work has held open a space in the field where contradiction, compassion, and precision can coexist. Your willingness to accompany this project, both symbolically and directly, has mattered more than I can say.

To Donnel Stern, for your intellectual generosity and early engagement with this material. Your work has shown how the unsymbolized can be held without forcing it to cohere too quickly—a principle that lives at the heart of this book.

To Christopher Bollas, Thomas Ogden, and Michael Eigen—your writings and generous feedback have helped contour the symbolic atmosphere of this project. I see this work as moving within a lineage you have each shaped—not by following, but by listening deeply to the textures of psychic life you helped make speakable.

To Phil Ringstrom, Ghislaine Boulanger, Susie Orbach, Salman Akhtar, and Aleksandra Wagner, for reading and responding to portions of this manuscript with care and thoughtfulness, and for the depth of presence you each bring to conversation. Your engagement supported the later stages of this work's formation in ways that continue to resonate.

To Donna Orange—your work helped make space for this voice to exist.

To my patients, whose psychic textures live between these lines—never exposed, but always shaping. Your presence informs this work in ways necessarily opaque, yet fundamentally constitutive.

To my husband, Tim—thank you for walking with me through the long arc of becoming. Your presence has steadied the inward work of finding my voice.

To those who shaped my early clinical formation—through training, supervision, and shared questioning — your impact remains, even when unspoken.

To a few trusted peers—including Mireille and Andrew—who held space for this thinking in its early, unsettled forms. Your presence at the edges of this work's emergence has mattered more than you know.

To Kate Hawes and Aakriti Aggarwal at Routledge, for your care and confidence in this project. And to the unnamed collective of readers, interlocutors, and co-dreamers who have helped this work take form across time and space—your traces are woven throughout.

This book is part of a larger project, *Unstable Objects*, whose arc continues to unfold.

If this book reaches you, may it find you where words falter—and remain with you there.

Preface—Recognition Reversal

When Knowing Undoes

"The instant I name, I estrange."
—after Derrida

I did not begin this book with a theory of absence. It arrived on the back of an ordinary analytic hour. A patient—call him Marcus—paused mid-sentence, eyes half closed, and whispered, "I feel known."

In that moment, his affect softened, almost dissolved, and what had been a pulsing current between us drained into a polite quiet. The recognition we had both longed for seemed to shut the room down. Something had been gained, but something—heat, danger, aliveness—was gone. I would meet the same hush, again and again, whenever a truth came too sharply into focus: the psyche flinches at illumination, folds itself inward, rewrites the scene.

I came to call this movement Recognition Reversal: the way psychic life is altered—and partially erased—by the very act of becoming knowable. Unlike repression, which hides before arrival, Recognition Reversal appears at the moment of finding. It is a twin birth: symbolization and undoing, presence and eclipse.

A Genealogy of the Reversal

The idea germinates in Derrida's *différance*, where any sign bears the trace of what it displaces; it echoes Laplanche's "enigmatic signifier," in which meaning is always in excess of itself; it riffs on Winnicott's paradox that the most intimate object is simultaneously created and found. But none of these lineages fully capture the clinical pulse: the lived micro-torsion in which a patient recognizes their rage, or longing, only to feel it evaporate; the therapist grasps a countertransference flash, only to watch it flatten when spoken.

Recognition Reversal reframes those moments as **structural, not incidental**. This book proposes that every act of psychic naming is accompanied by a reflexive curl—an undoing fold that both protects and depletes. Insight is never a simple acquisition; it is acquisition-plus-loss, revelation twinned with diminishment.

Why Begin Here?

Because this is a book about the seam where contact and collapse co-exist: each chapter explores a phenomenon—erotic submission, pathological accommodation, the "wise baby," the false self, the original paradox—in which psychic life surges forward *and* doubles back. Recognition Reversal is the red thread running through them all. Without it, the text might read as a catalogue of contradictions; with it, the contradictions disclose their architecture.

Clinical Texture

- **Marcus (Opening Silence):** The moment he felt *seen*, desire withdrew. Recognition Reversal framed this not as resistance, but as the psyche preserving opacity the instant it is endangered by visibility.
- **Eden (Erotic Submission):** When she named the pleasure of disappearing beneath a partner's will, her voice brightened—then grew technical, bloodless. The undoing did not negate her truth; it co-arose with it, signaling the cost of symbolizing what had thrived in the body's dusk.
- **Jonas (Pathological Accommodation):** Insight into his choreography of care laced him with relief and nausea. He laughed, called himself "textbook," and ceded the conversation to me. The insight survived only by partial self-erasure.

These moments are not failures of therapy; they are micro-demonstrations of how psyche and symbol grapple in real time. Throughout this book, you will see me lean *into* the reversal—sometimes letting the naming stand, other times allowing an unworded hum to protect what would recoil under light.

Theoretical Stakes

- **Derridean Trace:** Meaning is always already shadowed. Recognition Reversal introduces a clinical vector: the shadow moves in tandem with the speaker, conveying both concrete and affective aspects.
- **Laplanche and Translation:** Every translation distorts. Recognition Reversal asks: what psychic labor is accomplished *by* the distortion?
- **Bion and Transformation:** Alpha-function renders beta-elements thinkable; yet the newly coined alpha-elements can themselves disintegrate. The reversal is embedded in the apparatus.
- **Benjamin's Third:** Mutual recognition is fragile precisely because each party's subjectivity, once seen, risks becoming thing-like, losing elasticity.

A Note on Form

You will notice the chapters spiral rather than march. They return, revise, and unspool. This structure is intentional: the reader is invited to experience the very phenomenon under discussion. Recognition will arrive; reversal will follow; if we stay with both, something third—paradoxically steadier—may take shape.

How to Read What Follows

1. **Let yourself be undone.** If a passage clarifies, then cools, pause. That cooling is material.
2. **Track your counter-reading.** Where do you long for closure? Where do you resent its absence?
3. **Hold paradox as a method.** The text is built to hover between insight and unformulated knowing.

Acknowledgments of Unknowing

No preface can escape its own Recognition Reversal: in declaring the concept, I have already limited it. What follows may undo these pages; I hope it does. For now, let this be a prologue to unstable objects, unstable in part because the moment we meet them, they have begun to transform—or perhaps, begun to disappear.

Introduction

Holding What Cannot Be Healed

Psychoanalysis at the Edge

What if the psyche isn't a system to be understood, but a terrain to be witnessed? What if psychic truth is not hidden beneath defenses, waiting to be uncovered, but scattered across dissociation, enactment, and paradox—waiting instead to be held? This book begins at that edge. Not the edge of pathology or the edge of theory, but the edge where subjectivity begins to falter, fragment, and reform in the presence of another.

Unstable Objects traces a psychoanalysis attuned to those faltering moments: when feeling arrives out of time, when witnessing fails, when the self is performed rather than inhabited, when silence speaks more than speech. These are not failures of technique or structure; they are the very conditions under which psychic life can be reorganized—if someone is willing to stay close without requiring coherence. If classical psychoanalysis sought to decipher meaning through interpretation, this book aims to accompany meaning where it has not yet been formed. It turns toward the unformulated, the unsymbolized, the unclaimed.

Across its chapters, *Unstable Objects*—the book's conceptual subtitle—explores a field of analytic experience where dissociation is not just a defense, but a mode of communication; where submission is not surrender, but a reach toward relational re-entry; where paradox is not a logical impasse, but an ethical stance. The unstable object—whether patient, memory, symptom, fantasy, or theory—is not a problem to be solved but a phenomenon to be met. Psychoanalysis, in this light, becomes less about understanding the self and more about standing near the places where the self comes undone.

The title of the book reflects this stance. An unstable object is not broken—it is in motion. It flickers between forms, refusing reduction. Like many of the patients whose stories are woven through these pages, the unstable object demands a presence that does not interpret too quickly, a witnessing that does not resolve what cannot yet be lived. This is psychoanalysis not as a cure but as an *accompaniment*—a practice of staying close to what resists integration and loving it into symbol, time, and form.

DOI: 10.4324/9781003715283-1

Cartography of the Chapters

This book is not organized as a developmental arc. It does not move from surface to depth, symptom to core, or rupture to repair. Instead, it orbits a cluster of psychic phenomena—submission, secrecy, dissociation, foreclosure, paradox, and symbolic re-entry—each explored through its own chapter, but braided together by a shared sensibility: that psychic life is not linear and that healing does not always follow the path of integration.

The early chapters explore phenomena that shape psychic life from the margins:

- **"Secret Riverbeds: Secrecy and the Architecture of Subjectivity"** contends that secrecy is not simply a defense against exposure but a generative structure in the formation of self. It traces how secrets organize meaning, enact ethics, and silently structure the analytic field.
- **"Defenses Against Aliveness"** asks how shame, safety, and performance can become modes of self-inhibition. It explores how many patients defend not against trauma, but against contact—against the terrifying possibility of being felt and seen in real time.
- **"Erotic Submission and Fragmented Witnessing"** attends to the erotics of yielding—not as masochism, but as a dissociated choreography seeking repair. The submissive subject becomes legible not as a victim of perversion, but as a fragmented witness attempting to symbolize what was never metabolized.
- **"The Original Paradox"** traces the psychic legacy of early splitting and epistemic contradiction, drawing from Klein, Gödel, religious myth, and Derrida to argue that paradox is not a breakdown in development, but its substrate.

Later chapters deepen this ethos by tracing recurring motifs across clinical process, theory, and culture:

- **"The Madonna-Whore-Hologram"** rethinks erotic splitting as a form of self-fragmentation within gay male cruising culture, casting light on the recursive phantasies through which desire is dislocated and doubled.
- **"Ferenczi and the Dialectic of Coherence and Containment"** revisits *Confusion of Tongues*, not only as a trauma theory but also as a structural model for what happens when witnessing fails and containment inverts. This paper maps a dialectic: coherence as survival, containment as resurrection.
- **"The Wise Baby and the Unborn Self"** develops the figure of the prematurely knowing child—a psychic structure born not of growth but of foreclosure. Integrating Ferenczi, Winnicott, Bion, Heidegger, and Laplanche, the chapter explores what it means to survive by witnessing before one is witnessed.

- **"Time-Bound Selves: Curation, Collapse, and the Temporality of the False Self"** explores how the false self is not a mask, but a temporal structure that emerges when affect cannot unfold in time. Through clinical material and conceptual analysis, the chapter suggests that the false self curates coherence in the face of lived fragmentation.
- **"The False Self as Curator"** continues this exploration from a slightly different angle: how the curated self may not be false at all, but the most relationally developed form the subject has. Drawing from Winnicott, Foucault, and aesthetic theory, it rethinks the false/true binary as an ethical problem of belonging.
- **"Pathological Accommodation and the Architecture of Invisibility"** examines how patients survive by becoming what the other needs—structurally adapting to misrecognition. Drawing on Atwood, Stolorow, and Brandchaft, it contrasts interpretive working-through with relational rupture as the royal road to the real.

Each chapter stands alone, but together they form a constellation. Certain themes surface and resurface: the recursive nature of psychic time; the clinical labor of being-with rather than interpreting-too-soon; the intersubjective traces of secrecy, submission, and symbolic displacement; the affective residue that defies language but not encounter.

The chapters are not arranged in ascending theoretical density or narrative resolution. Rather, they gather and disperse, loop and return. The work of the book is not to progress toward clarity, but to dwell in fidelity to the unstable objects it honors.

The Subject Who Comes Too Soon

The subject of this book is not the cohesive ego, nor even the conflicted unconscious. It is the *unstable object*: the self who was used before it could emerge, whose early forms of recognition were always already misrecognitions, and who continues to carry the affective debris of relationships that never became symbolic. This subject does not seek to return to wholeness. It seeks to become liveable in paradox.

If psychoanalysis has long concerned itself with the structures that shape psychic life—drive, defense, symbolization, and intersubjectivity—*Unstable Objects* turns attention to structures that arrive prematurely, belatedly, or elliptically. These are selves formed too soon, witnessing before they were witnessed, signifying before they were held. They do not repress. They bypass. They survive not by splitting alone, but by becoming instruments in someone else's emotional architecture. These subjects do not simply lack integration—they were structured in absence, curated around invisibility.

We might call them after-subjects, or second-person selves. But perhaps it is better to follow Ferenczi and call them "wise babies": those who survived by adapting to the incoherence of the adult other, forming prematurely observing egos, stylized subjectivities, and false selves that are not masks but membranes—porous, responsive, chronically vigilant. They knew too much, too early, in order to be kept close. But they were not known.

The experience of the wise baby—like that of the erotically submissive patient, the pathologically accommodating self, or the queer subject formed through cultural abjection—is not one of simple trauma. It is the trauma of *symbolic substitution*: being used as a container before being a subject. These are not only patients who were hurt. They are patients who were overwritten. Their psyche is not a wound but a palimpsest—layered with the imprints of others' unmetabolized affect.

This book thus asks: what kind of psychoanalysis is required when we are not helping a patient return to their self, but helping a patient construct a self that was never permitted to form? What if the patient has been curating their visibility since infancy—subtly adapting their expression, sexuality, gender, performance, or even pain to keep the other emotionally intact? How do we work with dissociated subjectivity that does not want to be whole, but wants to be accompanied?

In this light, analytic work becomes less about coherence, more about co-presence. It becomes less a matter of interpretation than of witnessing. And the goal is not always integration, but *symbolic re-entry*—a second passage into life, made possible by a relational field that does not demand legibility or performance.

Each chapter in this book traces a version of that second passage: the erotic yielding that reclaims disavowed affect; the performance that hides a refusal to be known; the false self that protects the unborn; the analytic rupture that reorganizes more deeply than the interpretation. These are not resolutions. They are enactments of *arrival after the fact*—of becoming, not because the past is healed, but because something in the present can hold what the past foreclosed.

If there is a clinical ethic here, it is restraint. If there is a politics, it is of accompaniment over correction. And if there is a theory, it is one that follows affect before meaning, symbol before system, and paradox before coherence.

Paradox as Ontology

Psychoanalysis begins with splits—between conscious and unconscious, id and ego, self and object—but it is a paradox that most fully expresses the terrain of psychic life. Paradox is not contradiction. Contradiction demands resolution; paradox endures. It points to structures that cannot be reconciled, only inhabited. In this book, paradox is not simply thematic—it is ontological. It names the very mode of being of the unstable object: a subject formed through conditions that cannot be symbolically held without undoing their structure.

If the patient is both present and dissociated, both wave and particle, both knower and unformed, then no singular formulation will hold. Instead, the analytic stance must shift from understanding toward dwelling. We do not interpret the paradox. We take up residence within it. We sit with patients who simultaneously long to be seen and dread visibility, who crave merger but need distance, who offer symbolic gestures while foreclosing meaning. These are not neurotic conflicts. They are existential postures carved by survival.

Winnicott provides us with early language for this in his notion of transitional space—a third area between inner and outer reality where the child can play, imagine, and symbolize without collapse. But many patients never had access to such a space. Instead, they developed what I call *symbolic inversions*: using performance, sex, caretaking, or compliance to manage affect that could not be held symbolically. These inversions are paradoxical forms of contact: they represent what was foreclosed, often through enactment rather than insight.

To encounter such inversions clinically is to enter a zone where ordinary interpretation fails. The analyst must not solve the paradox but reverberate with it. This is what Thomas Ogden calls *reverie*—a state of analytic receptivity that allows unformulated experience to emerge between analyst and patient, often without immediate understanding. Or what Michael Eigen names the *feel of being*—a texture of emotional presence that is more primary than content.

Paradox, then, is not a problem to be solved, but the site of analytic work itself. It names the structure of early misrecognition and the possibility of symbolic re-entry. It organizes the patient's inner world and the analytic field. And when held without foreclosure, it becomes the medium through which new forms of selfhood may be tried, suffered, and endured.

In the chapters that follow, paradox appears in multiple forms: the false self that is more adaptive than the true, the erotic scene that enacts both surrender and agency, the analyst who must both witness and withhold. These are not theoretical puzzles. They are lived impasses. To work psychoanalytically at the edge of paradox is to accept that resolution may never come—and that something deeply human may still be forged in the effort to stay.

Dissociation, Temporality, and Symbolic Life

If paradox names the structure of experience, then dissociation names its temporal logic. Dissociation is not simply a defense; it is a way of organizing time. The dissociated self is not absent—it is elsewhere, displaced along a temporal axis that no longer unfolds linearly. The past is not past. Feeling is not anchored. The self appears in fragments, flashbacks, repetitions, or silences that do not align with narrative continuity. In this book, I take dissociation not as a clinical exception but as a default mode for many of the patients—and cultural moments—I write about.

Loewald reminds us that psychic life is fundamentally temporal. The ego does not emerge fully formed; it is constituted through a series of symbolizations that rework earlier experience into new relational forms. When this process is disrupted—by trauma, misattunement, or the foreclosure of affect—the symbolic function falters. Time no longer holds experience in sequence. Instead, affect and meaning are fragmented. Symbols recur not as integration but as residue.

This residue shows up in the consulting room as repetition compulsion, as muteness, as eroticized rituals, as recursive shame. It shows up in the analyst's countertransference as confusion, deadness, overinvolvement, or disorientation. These are not just resistances. They are indicators that time itself is not functioning as a medium of psychic life.

To address this, psychoanalytic work must become a form of temporal repair. Not by inserting the past into the present through interpretation, but by allowing the past to emerge in its unstructured form—what Ogden calls *undreamt dreams*—and slowly metabolizing it within the analytic field. The analyst does not restore time. They provide a rhythmic surround in which time might begin to flow.

Symbolic life, in this light, is not an abstract achievement. It is the capacity to hold experience in a temporally structured way. It is the difference between feeling and acting out, between memory and flashback, between word and symptom. When patients use fantasy, metaphor, or aesthetic form to symbolize previously unrepresentable states, they are not escaping reality—they are entering it. Symbolization is not a retreat from the real; it is its precondition.

Across the chapters of this book, symbolic life is explored not as an endpoint, but as a fragile and often deferred process. The wise baby, for instance, survives not through symbolization but through a premature knowing that forecloses play. The erotically submissive patient uses the body as a symbolic theater for disavowed affect. The analyst, in each case, must offer not just interpretation but presence—a capacity to sit with the nonlinear, the non-integrated, the temporally scrambled until something livable can emerge.

This is why aesthetic form matters. The writing itself must echo the temporal disruptions it describes. It must slow down, return, fragment, and hold silence. It must tolerate beauty and fracture in equal measure. Writing, like analysis, becomes a symbolic act that reorders dissociation—not into resolution, but into rhythm.

The Edge of Subjectivity: Where the Self Fails to Form

Each chapter in *Unstable Objects* traces an edge—where subjectivity flickers, where experience resists symbolization, where the analyst is drawn into relational fields that do not stabilize but tremble. These are not failures of treatment or signs of diagnostic pathology. They are encounters with the edge of what the self can bear.

In classical theory, the self is assumed to be a container of experience, capable of metabolizing affect and organizing relational life. But for many of the patients described in this book, the self is not a container. It is a threshold. A seam. A flicker. These patients are not organized around coherent defenses, but around holes—absences in the fabric of being that create not repression, but blankness. Dissociation is not their strategy; it is their ontology.

Ferenczi's work on the confusion of tongues provides a foundation here: when a child is required to bear what cannot be borne, they do not split between good and bad objects. They split between experience and selfhood. They know before they can feel. They survive without being. The self becomes a structure of substitution—there instead of someone else, for someone else, never quite for itself.

This structural absence reverberates across the book's figures: the prematurely observing child, the erotic submissive who feels only when used, the secretive self who stages symbolic life alone. Each exemplifies a form of subjectivity that is not false, but unstable—constructed in the absence of containment, organized through compensation, and animated by longing for a relational environment that never fully materialized.

The analytic task, in such cases, is not to interpret but to accompany. Not to fill in the gaps with theory, but to co-inhabit them. The analyst must learn to feel for the edges of presence—to sense when the patient is not there, or only partially there, or there for the analyst rather than for themselves. These are subtle forms of absence. They require a tolerance for uncertainty, for states that resist empathy because they are not being lived by the patient, only performed.

In this way, subjectivity itself becomes a paradox: something that can be present without being inhabited, enacted without being known. The self is not a stable center. It is a shifting field, often organized around others' needs, gazes, and failures. What remains is not the "true self" of Winnicott's vocabulary, nor the "false self" as a mask. What remains is a topology of absence—an architecture of unbeing around which experience must be delicately, symbolically, relationally re-formed.

This book moves through these edges not to repair them, but to dwell with them. To ask what kind of subjectivity can be built at the limits of being known. And what kind of psychoanalysis can survive—not in the face of fragmentation—but inside of it?

Methodology as Atmosphere: The Craft of Psychoanalytic Writing

In a discipline where theory often risks crystallizing into dogma and clinical experience into sanitized anecdote, the question of how to write psychoanalysis becomes as important as what to say. If *Unstable Objects* proposes a reframing of psychic life through paradox, recursive temporality, dissociation, and symbolic re-entry, then its methodology must itself reflect those dynamics. The form of the book is not merely a vehicle for its content—it is an enactment of it.

This section does not offer a technical manual. It offers, instead, a reflection on the craft of psychoanalytic writing as a relational act, an ethical discipline, and a form of aesthetic attunement. If these essays trace forms of emotional experience that often elude narrative integration—silence, secrecy, muteness, witnessing failure, states that arrive out of sequence—then the writing must remain capacious enough to hold such non-integration without collapse. Writing becomes a kind of containment, but a living one—not a coffin, but a cradle.

Psychoanalysis as a Literary Genre

Psychoanalytic writing exists in a strange hybrid genre: part philosophy, part science, part testimony, part literature. It is both clinical and speculative, personal and theoretical, bound by traditions and yet shot through with idiosyncrasy. As Adam Phillips has observed, the psychoanalytic case history has always had something of the novel in it—a narrative stitched from fragments, told with bias, textured by mood. And as Michael Eigen reminds us, psychoanalytic thought at its most vital is not a system, but a voice—a "tone of soul," a music that feels its way toward understanding without finalizing it.

In this book, I have tried to write in a voice that is neither omniscient nor confessional. Rather than present analysis as a polished theory or a resolved treatment, I try to capture the texture of working psychically in process—in the middle of contradiction, alongside fragments that speak but do not yet integrate. This is writing as accompaniment: not explanatory, but relational. Not to reduce the material into clarity, but to remain near its murk.

Countertransference as Method

Many of the chapters in *Unstable Objects* emerge from an atmosphere of countertransference—moments in which I, as analyst, found myself disoriented, flooded, compelled, or suspended. These are not simply reactions to the patient; they are data, feeling-states that enact the very psychic structures being explored. In the paper on erotic submission, for instance, the countertransference becomes a second body through which the patient's disavowed desire could begin to be metabolized. In the chapter on secrecy, the feeling of intellectual exclusion—of being "outside" what is being lived—was itself a re-enactment of the material's core logic.

I take seriously the invitation from theorists such as Donnel Stern and Thomas Ogden to treat countertransference not as noise to be filtered out, but as a terrain of meaning. This book does not claim neutrality. It is shaped by my own subjectivity as a clinician—by what I felt, feared, misread, endured, or longed for in the analytic field. The writing, then, becomes not a summary of experience, but an extension of it—a continuation of analytic listening into the realm of symbol and syntax.

Poetics and the Limits of Concept

Theory is essential to this work, but it is not sufficient. The phenomena explored here—fragmented desire, dissociative silence, symbolic enactment, recursive shame—are not easily captured in conceptual language. They resist it. They arrive before it, or after it, or outside it altogether. They require not only clinical precision, but a kind of lyricism—language that can hold emotional density without prematurely resolving it.

This is why many of the chapters use metaphors liberally. Not to mystify, but to reflect the fact that these psychic experiences are, by nature, analogical. A Klein bottle, a strange loop, a ghost limb, a suspended chord—these images do not explain the psyche, but they allow us to stay with what otherwise might slip away. They are not flights of fancy. They are containers for paradox.

But metaphor is not enough. At its worst, it risks aestheticizing trauma or obscuring the political conditions of psychic life. To write psychoanalytically is to move carefully between poetics and ethics—to let beauty arise where it serves the material, but never to substitute style for responsibility. This balance is especially important when writing about sexuality, trauma, or social vulnerability. What is tender must not be made shiny. What is raw must not be dressed up.

Chronology and Fragment

The organization of this book is not linear. It loops, revisits, and recasts. It begins in secrecy and ends in paradox, but each chapter could be read on its own or out of order. This is intentional. The psychic structures being explored—dissociation, foreclosure, recursive shame, symbolic re-entry—are themselves nonlinear. They resist coherent arcs. To write them linearly would be to betray their temporality.

Instead, I have structured the book more like a constellation. Each chapter takes a different angle on the unstable self—through myth, through the body, through witnessing, through language, through submission. Together, they create a psychic topology. The whole is not a system, but a field.

This also means the writing must tolerate gaps. Not every paradox is closed. Not every question is answered. This is not a flaw—it is fidelity to the experience. The unintegrated must sometimes remain unintegrated. The analyst does not always know. The writing must be willing to remain in that not-knowing long enough to allow something to emerge.

Toward an Analytic Aesthetic

What emerges, then, is not a method, but a kind of aesthetic. A way of writing that reflects the work of holding what cannot be healed, witnessing what cannot be spoken, and loving what cannot yet appear. If the analytic setting is a place where time can be reshaped, where paradox can be endured, then the writing of psychoanalysis must echo that temporality. It must slow down, circle back, pause, and reverberate. It must tolerate beauty and brokenness in equal measure.

In *Unstable Objects*, I try to write not only about psychoanalytic life, but from within it. The text itself becomes a holding environment—one that honors affective residue, symbolic texture, and psychic nonlinearity. In this way, I hope the reader feels not just informed, but accompanied.

Relational Lineage: On Gratitude and Ghosts

To write a book like *Unstable Objects* is also to write oneself into a lineage—of teachers, of texts, of conversations that shaped one's sensibility before one could name it. Though the book is composed of original chapters, each line carries the resonance of others: those I have studied with, those I have read, those I have loved, and those I have argued with in silence. Psychoanalysis is never practiced alone. It is relational not only in content but in inheritance.

This section is not an acknowledgments page. It is a reflection on the psychoanalytic and philosophical figures who haunt the pages of this book—not only as citations, but as presences. They have offered more than theory. They have offered a way of being with difficulty, a way of bearing the opacity of another's experience without needing to own or explain it. In that spirit, I want to briefly name the ghosts who have taught me how to listen.

The Clinicians

Hans Loewald gave me a language for time. His vision of psychoanalysis as a reorganization of psychic temporality—where the past can be symbolically re-animated in the present—underwrites nearly every chapter in this book. His notion that the analyst holds a "future" the patient has not yet lived makes therapeutic presence a metaphysical act.

Thomas Ogden taught me to think in the middle voice, to remain with what cannot yet be formulated, and to trust the process of dreaming the patient's undreamt dreams. His work invites not interpretation, but reverie.

Donnel Stern modeled how to think with both clarity and unknowing. His writing—especially on unformulated experience and the spontaneous emergence of meaning in dialogue—has shaped my clinical attention as much as my prose style.

Michael Eigen, perhaps more than anyone, gave me permission to write with affect. His work is less a system than a tone—a vulnerability that thinks, a sensibility that trembles, a form of scholarship that bleeds. This book is in deep conversation with its voice.

Nancy McWilliams, though her tone is more grounded, taught me that accessibility and depth are not in conflict. Her work on personality structure helped clarify how paradox inhabits not only states but entire character formations.

The Philosophers

Emmanuel Levinas stands behind this book like a silent sentinel. His notion of the ethical relation—of the self as summoned into being by the face of the other—saturates my understanding of subjectivity. He taught me that to be human is to be responsible, even before one is ready.

Michel Foucault haunts the chapters on surveillance, containment, and inscription. His analysis of power, knowledge, and the production of subjectivity frames much of how I understand psychic suffering—not as natural, but as historically and relationally organized.

Maurice Merleau-Ponty offered me a language for the body—not as object or shell, but as the site of lived meaning. His phenomenology taught me how the flesh gives rise to thought.

Ludwig Wittgenstein, with his quiet reflections on the limits of language, sits at the edge of nearly every page. "Whereof one cannot speak, thereof one must be silent"—and yet, we must try. That paradox is the ethos of this book.

Giorgio Agamben appears especially in the wise baby chapter, where his notions of the threshold figure—the sacred-excluded, the zone of indistinction—mirror the subject who is neither fully child nor adult, neither held nor exiled.

The Living and the Lost

Some of the figures who shaped me are alive and still writing. Others are no longer living, though their work continues to breathe in my sentences. Still others are not authors but patients, mentors, or friends. I write this book not only as a clinician, but as someone who has survived through the fragmentary coherence of analytic speech—through voices that steadied me and silences that called me to speak.

The chapters that follow are not monuments. They are correspondences. They carry traces of those I've read and those who have read me into being. I offer this section not as a formal homage, but as a whispered thank you—to those whose thinking has given shape to mine, and whose sensibility I hope to carry forward, not through imitation, but through fidelity to the work of staying close to what cannot yet be fully known.

Unstable Objects and the Shape of the Book

This book is composed of 11 chapters, each exploring a different terrain of psychic life where coherence frays and paradox becomes the only reliable compass. These chapters are not arranged to resolve into a linear arc but are constellated to form a recursive topology—a field of inquiry in which the reader may begin anywhere and return everywhere. The aim is not to build an argument, but to inhabit a rhythm: the rhythm of emergence, collapse, return, and reformation.

Each chapter stands alone, but all are joined by a shared orientation: a willingness to think with difficulty. This is a book about affective states that resist integration, truths that arrive out of sequence, and selves that cannot stabilize without distortion. And it is about how we, as analysts and as humans, bear witness to these phenomena—not to master them, but to accompany them.

Chapter Summaries

Chapter 1—Secret Riverbeds: Secrecy and the Architecture of Subjectivity

This chapter explores the psychic architecture of secrecy—not as defense or pathology, but as a fundamental structuring force in the formation of selfhood. Drawing on Ferenczi, Loewald, Bollas, and Derrida, this examination explores how withheld experience can shape the inner world as a kind of subterranean current, influencing symbolic life from below.

Chapter 2—Defenses Against Aliveness: Safety, Shame, and the Inhibition of Contact

This chapter considers how certain forms of psychic safety—especially those organized around perfectionism, self-effacement, or intellectualization—may defend against the unbearable intensity of contact. Drawing on Winnicott, Panksepp, Benjamin, and Merleau-Ponty, it reframes inhibition not as pathology but as a developmental compromise that protects the sWelf from annihilation by feeling.

Chapter 3—Erotic Submission and Fragmented Witnessing

This chapter examines erotic submission not as masochism or regression, but as a symbolic site where fragmented desires and disavowed longings can be enacted, witnessed, and—at times—held. Drawing on Laplanche, Jessica Benjamin, Bersani, Klein, and Edelman, it traces how submission can offer a return to affective states that were never metabolized in a relationship.

Chapter 4—The Original Paradox: Splitting, Symbolization, and the Birth of the Subject

This chapter explores paradox as the original structure of psychic life—tracing its lineage from creation myths and Klein's positions through Gödel's incompleteness theorems and Derridean *différance*. It frames paradox not as a failure of thought, but as the very form through which the psyche maintains internal complexity without collapse.

Chapter 5—The Madonna–Whore–Hologram: Erotic Idealization and Internal Fracture

This chapter considers the split between sexualization and tenderness—especially in gay male relational life—as a structure of internal division shaped by fantasy, projection, and traumatic relational history. The "hologram" is introduced as a third mode of psychic engagement, where contradiction can be held without splitting.

Chapter 6—Ferenczi: The Dialectic of Coherence and Containment

This chapter revisits Ferenczi's *Confusion of Tongues* through the clinical dialectic between coherence and containment. Drawing on Bollas, Laplanche, Ogden, and Orange, it reframes the analytic task not as restoring narrative, but as creating a symbolic surround where affect may emerge before it can be understood.

Chapter 7—The Wise Baby and the Unborn Self

This chapter explores the prematurely knowing child—the "wise baby"—as a developmental structure marked by dissociation, inverted witnessing, and foreclosure of affect. It links clinical material to myth, logic, quantum theory, and embodiment, suggesting that analytic repair involves not insight but rebirth into a symbolic field that was never first formed.

Chapter 8—Time-Bound Selves: Curation, Collapse, and the Temporality of the False Self

This chapter investigates the temporal dimensions of the false self, arguing that it functions not simply as a defensive mask but as a curator of psychic time. It examines how the false self preserves continuity by organizing affective life into sequences that can be tolerated and how this temporal scaffolding both protects and limits the aliveness of the subject.

Chapter 9—The False Self as Curator: Structure, Survival, and the Ethics of Performance

Building on Winnicott, this chapter reframes the false self as a structure of ethical survival—a curated relational artifact that performs the conditions under which the subject was permitted to exist. It explores the tension between vitality and adaptation, presence and curation, and asks whether the false self can become a site of creative reformation rather than a symptom of alienation.

Chapter 10—The Original Paradox, Revisited

This chapter circles back to the theme of paradox through Klein, Freud, and creation myth, exploring how early psychic division gives rise to symbolic life. It considers the paradoxical truth that the self is always already split and that this split is the source of both suffering and creativity. The chapter closes by reframing psychoanalysis not as integration, but as a practice of staying near the edges of coherence with enough presence to let something new be born.

Chapter 11—Pathological Accommodation and the Architecture of Invisibility

This chapter explores pathological accommodation as a psychic strategy organized around anticipatory erasure. It traces how the self becomes invisible through the preservation of others' coherence and how analytic rupture can expose a more saturated, drive-laden core that resists symbolic integration.

An Invitation

Unstable Objects is not a book that moves toward synthesis. It lingers in fragmentation. It honors the rhythms of dissociation, the dignity of the provisional, and the beauty of truths that arrive before they can be lived. It is written in the hope that psychoanalysis might continue to expand its reach—not by becoming more totalizing, but by becoming more capacious. Not by resolving contradiction, but by making space for it.

In that spirit, I invite the reader not to read this book straight through, but to circle with it. To begin where they feel drawn. To let what doesn't yet make sense hang in the air. And to listen for the reverberations of their own unstable objects—those fragments of aliveness that, when held with care, begin to speak.

Part 1

Hidden Structures and Symbolic Terrain

1 Secret Riverbeds

Secrecy and the Architecture of Subjectivity

Secrecy is a foundational yet underexamined dimension of psychic life. Reflecting on sexual secrecy, the existential closet, and the embodied life of the unsaid, this chapter explores how hidden truths and private experiences shape subjectivity, interpersonal fields, and bodily symptomatology. Drawing on psychoanalytic theory, clinical vignettes, and continental philosophy, secrecy is reframed as a paradox: both a protective sanctuary and a source of isolation. Psychoanalytic treatment becomes a space where secrets may be reverently witnessed rather than prematurely revealed. In attending to these *secret riverbeds*, the psychoanalyst honors what remains hidden while fostering the possibility of relational contact and psychic transformation.

Introduction

Every psyche harbors secrets. Unspoken experiences, forbidden desires, shameful memories, and untold stories form subterranean streams flowing beneath the surface of everyday life. These hidden currents carve out channels—secret riverbeds within the architecture of subjectivity—tracing the unseen patterns that shape how we become who we are. What is kept secret (from others and even from oneself) can subtly influence how a person feels, behaves, and connects. Our secrets shape our lives much like the underground rivers quietly determine the landscape above.

From its inception, psychoanalysis has been preoccupied with secret undercurrents. It viewed the human subject as structured in such a way that hidden truths seek expression through indirect means. Early in his work, Sigmund Freud viewed neurotic symptoms as the result of repressed painful experiences or unacceptable wishes pushed out of awareness yet continuing to exert influence. The cases of Dora (Freud, 1953a) and Little Hans (Freud, 1955a) hinge on what was not said. Dora's unexplained coughs and silences become emissaries of the unspeakable—carrying veiled sexual knowledge and familial intrigue. Little Hans's childhood phobia is entwined with a "secret" theory of where babies come from. Freud initially believed that uncovering a traumatic secret (an early sexual seduction) would cure

DOI: 10.4324/9781003715283-3

hysterical symptoms, a view revised as he recognized the role of fantasy and desire.

Nonetheless, the fundamental idea remained: psychic life abounds with hidden chambers and passageways; bringing the contents of these spaces into the light shared by a clinician and a patient is a path toward healing. In Freud's structural model, the unconscious itself is a vault of secrets, filled with wishes and memories kept from consciousness by the ego's defenses. Psychoanalytic therapy thus became an archaeology of the unconscious—a careful excavation of the material winding beneath the patient's conscious narratives.

Secrecy is not solely a matter of pathology or something to be eliminated from psychic life. This paper deals with *the paradox of secrecy*: while some secrets fester and imprison the self, others provide a necessary refuge for individuality. D. W. Winnicott (1965) captured this paradox eloquently when he wrote, "it is joy to be hidden but disaster not to be found" (p. 186). The capacity to hold something privately is as vital to the self as the need to be recognized. Yet, the world made of secrets can also feel as an imprisonment. Winnicott goes on to note that *"each individual is an isolate, permanently non-communicating, permanently unknown, in fact unfound"* (p. 187, emphasis in the original). In his view, every person retains an inner sanctum—an "unfound" self—never fully accessible, even in the deepest intimacy.

Such ideas point to secrecy as an essential component of subjectivity, not merely a neurotic aberration. Indeed, subjectivity may be imagined as a house of many rooms—some open and sunlit, others shadowed, with a few concealed chambers known only to the self. The question then is not whether to abolish secrecy, but how its presence shapes the self's development and its relations with others. When does a secret become a protective inner sanctuary, and when does it turn into a prison of isolation or source of psychopathology?

To address these questions, I aim to integrate multiple perspectives. Classical psychoanalytic theorists like Freud and Melanie Klein provide a foundation for understanding how secrets operate in intrapsychic life (for example, through repression or splitting). Post-Freudian object relations theorists such as W. R. D. Fairbairn and Harry Guntrip deepen this understanding by describing internal worlds populated by secret imagos and hidden self–other interactions. Their work on schizoid phenomena portrays individuals who live more fully in a rich inner world of fantasy than in the visible outer world of relationships. In parallel, existential philosophers and dialogical thinkers—Martin Buber, Emmanuel Levinas, Martin Heidegger—offer insights into the role of secrecy in human existence. They remind us that not all that is meaningful can be said: the Other always retains an unknowable alterity (Levinas, 1969); truth involves a dynamic of **concealment and unconcealment** (Heidegger, 1962); a genuine encounter requires openness yet acknowledges the "between" space that cannot be fully articulated (Buber, 1970). These philosophical viewpoints help us consider secrecy not just as a feature of individual psychology, but as a fundamental aspect of being-in-the-world and relating to others.

The Role of Secrecy in the Formation of Subjectivity

I will explore several key dimensions of the role of secrecy in the formation of subjectivity. One section begins with theoretical foundations in psychoanalysis, examining how the unconscious internal object relations create a structural architecture of secrecy within the psyche. The next section delves into sexual secrets and *the existential closet*, analyzing how identities and desires kept hidden (sexual orientations, infidelities, or paraphilias) impact one's sense of authenticity and being. This section integrates themes of shame and revelations of individuals' secrets with clinical vignettes illustrating living in closets, both literal and metaphorical. The following section focuses on the embodiment of secrecy: how secrets live in the body. Drawing on Wilhelm Reich's (1949) concept of body armor, I consider cases where unspoken trauma or emotion is expressed through physical symptoms—how the body "speaks" the secret language of the unconscious. The next section discusses relational architectures of secrecy in families, couples, and the therapeutic relationship. Here, I rely on Harry Stack Sullivan's (1953) interpersonal approach, contemporary relational psychoanalysis, particularly the work of Stephen Mitchell (1988), and intersubjective systems theory (Stolorow et al., 2002) to understand how secrets shape and are shaped by relational dynamics. What happens in the space between people when truth is withheld? How do secret-keeping and revelation of secrets influence intimacy, trust, and the co-construction of reality in a relationship or in therapy?

I then turn to clinical implications and the dialectic of hiding versus revealing within the therapeutic setting and discuss the techniques and challenges in working with secrets. This work demands creation of a safe space where patients can gradually bring forth long-held secrets (traumatic histories or deeply shameful wishes); negotiation of the timing of interpretations or disclosures; and respect for the patient's right to privacy versus the therapeutic value of honesty. Throughout, clinical vignettes illustrate how a skilled navigation of secrecy—honoring its protective function while mitigating its isolating effects—can facilitate transformation. The synthesis of these insights suggests that secrecy is both a structural necessity in the formation of subjectivity and a dynamic process to be worked with in therapy. One section explores how this theoretical inquiry, centered on psychoanalytic and Western philosophical traditions, is countered by a proposal for future directions such as cross-cultural studies of secrecy, links with attachment theory and neuroscience, and further integration of philosophical ideas—to enrich psychoanalytic conceptions of the unseen forces shaping our lives.

By weaving together psychoanalytic nuance, philosophical resonance, and clinical texture, I aim to illuminate the secret riverbeds that wind beneath our lives, moving beyond a view of secrets as impediments to cure. Instead, secrets are viewed as fundamental elements in the architecture of the self—ranging from the poisonous to the profound. By weaving together psychoanalytic nuance, philosophical depth, and clinical experience, I hope to illuminate the secret riverbeds that run within us and to guide therapists in navigating this terrain toward healing and authentic connection.

Foundations: The Psychic Architecture of Secrecy

Psychoanalysis was born from the revelation of secrets. In the late 19th century, Freud's patients—Anna O. and later Dora—found relief from hysterical symptoms when long-buried secrets were spoken aloud. In Freud's and Josef Breuer's early cathartic method, the act of conveying a traumatic secret was likened to draining an abscess: the pressure of the unsaid was released, and the symptom often abated. This gave rise to the first topography of the mind, dividing it into the conscious (accessible thoughts), the preconscious (potentially accessible memories), and the unconscious (the sequestered repository of repressed secrets). The unconscious, in Freud's formulation, is not a storehouse but an actively guarded vault. The mind's architecture includes censoring mechanisms (primarily repression) that keep certain ideas out of awareness because they threaten the stability of the conscious ego. Thus, the psyche is structurally built to have secrets; repression ensures that some content remains hidden even from the self. Slips and dream symbols demonstrate how the hidden contents seek expression in disguise. A patient might forget the name of a person who is the object of a forbidden love, or dream of muddy water when harboring a shameful experience—both indirect signs of what Freud called "the return of the repressed," the secret attempting to surface.

Freud's view of secrecy was dynamic: the secret presses for discharge and finds a way out through symptoms, parapraxes, or somatic leakage. He recognized that the body itself could betray secrets that the mind refuses to utter. In *Fragment of an Analysis of a Case of Hysteria* (1953/1905), commenting on Dora's nervous fiddling with her purse, Freud remarked that "He that has eyes to see and ears to hear may convince himself that no moral can keep a secret. If his lips are silent, he chatters with his finger-tips; betrayal oozes out of him at every pore" (*SE* 7, pp. 77–78). Here Freud elegantly conveys that the human organism is an open system: psychic secrets inevitably seek communicative outlets, often through the body's gestures and symptoms. This will resonate later with Reich's notion of organismic truth in the body but, even at the outset, Freud observed that hidden mental content finds its voice somatically. Secrecy, then, is a psychophysiological process.

Another aspect Freud highlighted is the interpersonal dimension of secrets in therapy: the neurotic individual is often keeping secrets both from self and from the analyst (and originally, from parental figures). The fundamental rule of psychoanalysis, free association, is essentially an injunction against secrecy in the consulting room. Freud realized that patients often resist this rule; they feel embarrassment or fear revealing certain thoughts. This resistance is itself evidence of the power of secrecy in psychic life. The analyst's task is to gently overcome the resistance, creating an atmosphere of non-judgment so that previously unspeakable thoughts can be voiced. Freud likened the analyst to an archaeologist digging through layers of a ruin: each layer of narrative and memory might conceal deeper strata, and the true meaning of a symptom might lie at the buried psychic core.

While Freud emphasized individual secrets and the uncovering of specific hidden contents, later psychoanalytic thinkers extended the concept of secrecy to the very structure of the self. Melanie Klein, working with young children, observed that even toddlers have rich internal lives with secrets in the form of *unconscious phantasies*. In Klein's theory, from infancy onward the mind contains internal objects that are not directly shared. A child in the paranoid-schizoid position, for example, might secretly harbor aggressive fantasies toward the "bad" breast while outwardly cooing at the real mother. Klein showed that children use splitting and projective identification as mechanisms that both reveal and conceal inner truth. If a toddler projects their angry feelings into a doll and then scolds the doll, the actual rage at the parent remains a kind of secret, displaced onto a toy. The caregiver might see the outburst toward the doll but fail to realize that it encodes a message about the child's internal state. Thus, from a Kleinian perspective, the mind's architecture includes partitions: aspects of the self (and representations of others) are segregated to maintain an image of the good self and good object uncontaminated by badness. They correspond to what Klein (1946) called "internal psychic reality," a realm often quite distinct from what the individual shows publicly. Klein's later work on envy and gratitude (1975) can also be read through the lens of secrecy: envy, too, might be kept as a shameful secret, because to admit it would threaten the relationship with the other.

Klein's British object relations successors made the notion of a "secret inner world" even more explicit. W. R. D. Fairbairn reconceptualized libido (psychic energy) not as pleasure-seeking, but as seeking relationships. He argued that, when external relationships disappoint or injure the child, the child withdraws libido from outer reality and invests it in internal object relations. In doing so, the child internalizes the bad and good figures and related aspects of self, creating an internal drama that can be largely hidden from view. Fairbairn's model of the psyche divides the ego into parts: a central ego linked with an ideal object (the loved, good part) and split-off structures—the libidinal ego attached to an exciting but unsatisfying object and the anti-libidinal (or internal saboteur) ego attached to a rejecting object. This complex internal trio amounts to a secret theatre of the mind: a person might consciously present as friendly and normal, while unconsciously they are caught in a painful relationship with internalized bad objects while maintaining a secret longing for an idealized figure. Fairbairn (1952) actually emphasized the element of secrecy in schizoid personalities: such individuals appear emotionally detached or bland, but internally they often guard a rich imaginative life, sometimes populated by what he termed "illusory relationships" with internal objects. This inner life is kept secret because it feels safer and more gratifying than any connection with real others, especially if they have been unreliable or hurtful.

Extending Fairbairn, Harry Guntrip (1969) described the schizoid retreat into an inner world in poignant terms. He portrayed some patients as living in a "laboratory" of the self—a controlled inner environment where they are beholden only to their own fantasies and internal figures, while externally they may play a role of normalcy or remain distant. Guntrip noted that these individuals often have a secret self that was never shared or validated in childhood; as adults they preserve this true self in isolation, sometimes presenting a *false self* to the world. Here we see secrecy as a protective strategy: the most intimate, vulnerable core of the self goes into hiding because exposure felt life-threatening in early relationships. The secret self becomes like a hermit in a cave; safe from harm, but also alone.

Winnicott (1965) similarly described how an infant might comply with the parents' expectations by developing a *false self*, while the *true self* remains hidden and unarticulated. He comments directly on secrecy: "We can understand the hatred people have of psych-analysis which has penetrated a long way into the human personality, and which provides a threat to the human individual in his need to be secretly isolated" (1965, p. 186). The capacity to hide something (the *true self* or a creative impulse) and to reveal it in symbolic form (art, play, or selected interpersonal moments) is crucial to healthy development. Thus, object relations theory paints the architecture of subjectivity as fundamentally two-layered: an outward-facing self that engages in social reality and an inward-facing self that dwells in a private world of objects and fantasies. Whereas every person has some degree of inner life that is private, pathology enters when the bridge between inner and outer breaks down—when the inner world becomes a locked vault with the person trapped inside, or, conversely, when the inner world is so disavowed that the person loses authenticity.

It is important to note that secrecy, in this context, refers to the structure, the way the psyche organizes experience such that some aspects are deliberately not communicated or even consciously acknowledged. Even the classical Freudian superego can be thought of as a secret agency within the self: it observes and judges the ego often outside of awareness, keeping its own counsel of harsh criticisms or ideals. Often we are only dimly aware of how severely we judge ourselves internally; that harshness might be a secret carried from a punitive parent now living on in the superego. Similarly, the Freudian id—*a cauldron of wishes and impulses*—operates largely in secret, revealing itself only in disguised fashion through dreams and slips. Thus the structural model can be read as a blueprint of secret compartments within the mind (id, ego, superego), with the ego acting as a kind of executive that decides what secrets to keep or reveal.

Beyond individual structure, secrecy also has a developmental trajectory. Having secrets is a normal part of development. Children have imaginary friends, secret clubs, diaries with locks, and hideouts. Developmental psychologists note that forming secrets can aid the emergence of a sense of self distinct from parents. A child who whispers with a friend or keeps a private diary is experimenting with autonomy and identity. Psychoanalytically, this resonates with Mahler et al.'s (1975) separation–individuation process: the child stepping away from merger with the caregiver, carving out a private mental space. Too little space afforded secrecy (an intrusive parent who invades the child's every thought) can stunt the child's individuation; too much secrecy (a child forced to keep family traumas in silence) can overburden the child and lead to psychopathology.

Thus, a balance is needed. Masud Khan (1974) wrote about the "privacy of the self," arguing that an individual requires a private domain of experience that has to be respected if healthy psychological growth is to occur. He suggested that therapy must respect certain secrets or privacy that a patient maintains, rather than forcing disclosure of everything. This is a nuanced counterpoint to the classical Freudian push for total frankness. Sometimes, keeping a secret can be adaptive, allowing a sense of control or dignity. An adolescent might not want to share his nascent sexual fantasies with parents or even with a therapist immediately; respecting that boundary can be crucial for their developing sense of agency. Khan and Winnicott both caution that there is a right to one's own secret life, a portion of experience that can remain unspoken yet still known and validated indirectly through the therapeutic relationship.

As we have seen, the psychic architecture of secrecy is multi-layered. At the deepest level, the unconscious itself is a realm of hidden truth where repression hides what the conscious mind cannot bear; at the level of object relations, the personality may be divided into inner vs. outer selves that hold secrets from each other and from the world; and developmentally, the formation of a private inner world is both normal and essential. Classical analysis sought to illuminate the darkness of the unconscious, bringing secrets into speech to relieve symptoms. Later perspectives acknowledge that some darkness is intrinsic to being human: an "unfound" element of self might never be fully communicable.

The task of psychoanalytic understanding, then, is not to eradicate secrecy but to discern its role in each individual's psychic economy. What secrets does this person keep and why? How do these secret riverbeds underlie their conscious life? Are the secret psychic chambers filled with terrifying ghosts (traumatic memories, persecutory objects) that need the light of day, or are they protective shelters housing the tender, creative aspects of self that have not yet found a safe relational home?

Sexual Secrecy and the Existential Closet

Sexuality and secrecy are intimately entwined. From Freud's earliest case studies to contemporary queer theory, psychoanalytic thought has repeatedly reflected on how erotic life is shaped by what must be hidden, fantasized, or only partially expressed. Sexual secrecy often begins long before a specific act or identity is formulated; it emerges as a structural aspect of subjectivity, particularly when sexual desires or identifications deviate from social norms.

Freud's account of infantile sexuality already presumes an atmosphere of secrecy: the child's polymorphous perversity must eventually be repressed and redirected into socially acceptable adult sexuality. The Oedipus complex is an inescapable psychic drama that requires repression to create a normative adult identity. In Freud's view, civilization demands that these primal sexual wishes remain largely unconscious; the cultural superego builds a world atop forbidden loves and secret resentments. Thus, even the most "normal" adult is a carrier of unacknowledged erotic secrets.

For queer individuals, secrecy becomes even more constitutive. In societies organized around heteronormative expectations, gay, lesbian, bisexual, transgender, and queer individuals grow up absorbing an implicit (and often explicit) message that their desires are unspeakable, shameful, dangerous, or invisible. In her magisterial work, *Epistemology of the Closet* (1990), Eve Kosofsky Sedgwick argues that the very structure of modern sexual identities depends on a public/private split: certain truths must be managed, hidden, disclosed strategically, or never acknowledged at all. Sedgwick extends psychoanalytic thinking by suggesting that the "closet" is not merely a psychological defense but a structure shaping subjectivity.

My own work with gay men reveals how the existential closet is not only a historical artifact of a more homophobic past, but a deep ontological structure. One patient, a successful professional in his forties, comfortably "out" in most areas of his life, struggled with persistent feelings of unreality and fraudulence. In analysis, he described how, as a child, long before he knew what "gay" meant, he felt a visceral sense that some core aspect of himself must remain hidden in order for him to survive. He recalled sitting at the family dinner table and sensing a need to "mask" or "pass" even though no one had accused him of anything. His secret was not yet a specific act or identity; it was an unnameable difference, an ineffable "otherness" that required cloaking.

This clinical vignette illustrates and confirms that secrecy precedes content. It is not that the child has a secret he consciously chooses to keep. Rather, the atmosphere into which he is born demands concealment. R. D. Laing's (1960) descriptions of ontological insecurity—a sense of being exposed, invaded, or annihilated if one's authentic self were fully seen—also indicate that, to survive, the self must create false fronts; not out of deception, but out of existential necessity.

Martin Buber's distinction between I-Thou and I-It relations sharpens this clinical point. In a world that meets the emergent gay self as an It—an object to be scrutinized, judged, or punished—the subject must protect the nascent Thou within. The gay child learns, often without explicit instruction, that direct self-revelation is perilous. Thus, secrecy is not a *post hoc* defense against a specific threat; it is a structural precondition for survival in a hostile or indifferent world.

Emmanuel Levinas's ethics of alterity further deepens this line of understanding. Levinas insists that the Other is not to be assimilated into the Same; the opacity of the Other must be respected. In this light, the gay child's secrecy may be seen as an ethical preservation of their alterity in the face of a world that would otherwise flatten or erase it. From a clinical standpoint, this reframes "coming out" not as a confession or a disclosure, but as a profoundly ethical negotiation: when, how, and with whom is one's hiddenness relinquished?

The existential closet also leaves bodily traces. Patients often describe chronic vigilance, hyper-attunement to others' perceptions, and somatic symptoms like muscle tension, gastrointestinal distress, or insomnia—all signs of the embodied labor of secrets-keeping. The closet lives in the body long after a person has cognitively embraced their sexual identity. These bodily imprints must be addressed in therapy through an attuned witnessing of the patient's somatic language.

Clinical work with sexual secrecy thus demands patience, humility, and an acceptance of opacity. Analysts must resist the temptation to rush toward disclosure. The act of speaking a secret prematurely, before it has ripened in the patient's inner world, can be retraumatizing. Conversely, respecting the pace at which secrets unfold—and sometimes allowing them to remain partially hidden—can enable deeper trust and integration.

One striking example comes from a gay male patient who spent several years in analysis before revealing that he had a longstanding practice of anonymous sexual encounters in public spaces. The revelation came gradually in fragments and hesitations. When he finally articulated these experiences, my non-intrusive curiosity allowed the patient to explore the complex mix of shame, excitement, longing, and autonomy that had structured his sexuality. Importantly, the patient's disclosure did not lead to an interpretation of pathology; it was approached as an essential expression of self that had been hidden both from others and from parts of himself.

Thus, sexual secrecy—and the broader phenomenon of the existential closet—reflects the intimate architecture of hiddenness within subjectivity. Secrecy here is neither wholly pathological nor wholly protective; it is a riverbed along which eros, identity, and survival have had to flow.

Embodied Secrecy: The Body as a Secret Archive

Secrecy lives not only in language and mind but also in the body. The hidden tensions, unrevealed traumas, and unspoken affects that structure psychic life are often inscribed somatically. Wilhelm Reich's early work offers foundational insights into how the body becomes a secret archive of unprocessed experience.

Reich (1949) argued that chronic muscular tension—what he termed *character armor*—is a bodily manifestation of repressed emotion and unexpressed truths. The tight jaw, the rigid pelvis, the shallow breathing: these are not random physical habits but psychodynamic strategies for holding back rage, grief, terror, or longing. The body holds what the psyche cannot yet face. In psychoanalytic work, attending to the patient's bodily language—the sudden tightening, the flutter of fingers, the averting of gaze—can reveal secrets that words cannot yet carry.

A patient who carries a secret of early sexual abuse, for instance, might display a persistent slouching posture, as if trying to make herself invisible. Another patient who harbors secret rage at a neglectful parent may suffer from chronic migraines, the mind-body system attempting to compress forbidden aggression into somatic symptomatology.

Otto Rank's notion of birth trauma adds another layer to the embodiment of secrecy. Rank (1929) proposed that the existential anxiety of separation from the maternal body leaves an indelible mark on subjectivity—a memory of loss and rupture that shapes all subsequent attachments. From this perspective, the body carries pre-verbal secrets: unformulated experiences of abandonment, yearning, terror, and desire that precede linguistic representation.

Michael Eigen's work deepens the psychoanalytic understanding of embodied secrecy and psychic withdrawal. In *The Psychotic Core* (1986), he describes how "the stupor that once relieved [the infant] in face of catastrophe becomes part of a debilitating attempt at self-repair or, finally, a giving up, a lapse into unintegration" (p. 122). This form of disappearance—more primitive than denial—arises from what he calls "an elemental response to agony," where "we are all marked by dead or numb spots that, at the deepest levels, bear witness to a loss or lapse of existence that once seemed endless" (p. 122). In the clinical setting, such dissociative blanking out may not be verbally expressed but instead surface through posture, affect, or the collapse of vitality. The analyst's task is to stay near this inner silence, to receive its gravity without rushing toward coherence, and to tolerate, as Eigen puts it, "the most ghastly horror and the saving bliss" (p. 122) that accompany the psyche's repeated return from its own edges.

In clinical practice, honoring embodied secrecy means listening not only to the patient's narratives but to their somatic expressions of what cannot yet be told. It requires cultivating a reverie that allows the analyst's own body to register the patient's unspoken truths—an embodied countertransference that senses the riverbeds of hidden life flowing beneath the analytic dialogue.

A patient chronically laughed when discussing painful topics. Instead of interpreting the laughter as mere resistance, the analyst sensed in her own chest a constriction, a pressure to exhale emotion that the patient could not yet release. Holding this embodied awareness allowed a different kind of listening—one that eventually enabled the patient to feel the sorrow that had been contained within the armor of laughter.

Thus, the body serves both as a guardian of secrets and a gateway to their eventual emergence. Recognizing and respecting the body's role deepens the psychoanalytic encounter, allowing therapy to reach dimensions of the self that verbal interpretation alone cannot access.

Relational Architectures of Secrecy: The Space Between

Secrecy is profoundly relational. Secrets emerge, are maintained, and are revealed within interpersonal fields. The analytic situation is a privileged arena where secrets are negotiated—sometimes spoken, sometimes silently preserved, and often enacted in subtle ways between analyst and patient.

Harry Stack Sullivan's interpersonal theory offers a crucial foundation for understanding secrecy relationally. Sullivan (1953) posited that the self is constituted through patterns of relating—what he called "personifications" and "self-systems"—designed to manage anxiety. Within this framework, secrecy is not a hiding from the other but a mutual negotiation of what can be shown and seen. Certain aspects of the self are kept secret because the relational field (family, culture, society) cannot accommodate them without inducing annihilating shame or anxiety. Thus, secrecy arises from the relational imperative to survive emotionally in a particular human environment.

Stephen Mitchell further elaborates how self-experience is co-constructed in dynamic interpersonal contexts. In *Relational Concepts in Psychoanalysis* (1988), he emphasized that identities and experiences are co-created in real time within relationships; they are not merely pre-existing entities hidden within the self. Secrets are not static possessions but relational phenomena. They are aspects of experience that emerge or are suppressed depending on the interpersonal matrix in which the subject moves.

In the clinical encounter this means that what a patient reveals—or cannot reveal—is profoundly influenced by the relational stance of the analyst. An atmosphere of intrusive curiosity, premature interpretation, or covert moral judgment can re-enact the very conditions that made secrecy necessary. Conversely, an atmosphere of attuned reverie, respectful pacing, and acknowledgment of the patient's right to privacy can create the conditions under which long-held secrets may find expression.

Stolorow, Brandchaft, and Atwood's intersubjective systems theory (1987) offers a further refinement. They argue that experience is always co-constituted within affective systems involving self and other. When the subject's affective states are not validated or mirrored, the ensuing traumatic experience leads to a retreat into secrecy and isolation. Thus, therapy must focus not on uncovering secrets as isolated facts but on reweaving the affective fabric in which the secret became necessary.

After years of analytic work, a female patient disclosed that she had been carrying a secret about her parentage—she had learned as a teenager that the man who raised her was not her biological father. Her initial disclosure was not verbal; it was enacted in the analytic field through a prolonged period of confusion, missed appointments, and apparent resistance. When the patient finally found the words to articulate her secret, it became clear that the analyst's patient tolerance of the nonverbal enactments—without intrusive demand for explanation—had created the necessary holding environment for disclosure.

Secrecy is thus not a static possession to be "extracted" by the analyst but a dynamic element of the relational field. The secret may live in silences, somatic expressions, gaps in the narrative, or the analyst's own countertransference experiences of confusion, distance, or pressure.

Adam Phillips's reflections on secrecy, mystery, and the ethics of non-knowledge further inform this clinical stance. In *On Flirtation* (1994), Phillips suggests that preserving mystery is essential to vitality and desire. Over-interpretation and the analytic compulsion to know everything can deaden the analytic encounter. Sometimes the deepest respect for the patient's subjectivity lies in allowing what remains secret to remain partially veiled, at least for a time.

Thus, in psychoanalytic work, engaging with secrecy relationally requires a stance of ethical humility: the willingness to accompany the patient along their secret riverbeds without necessarily demanding to drain them.

Working with Secret Riverbeds: Clinical Implications

The delicate clinical task when working with secrecy requires balancing the tension between interpretation and reverence, between encouraging disclosure and respecting the sanctity of hiddenness.

First, analysts must recognize that not all secrets are pathogenic. Some secrets protect fragile aspects of selfhood that are not yet ready for relational exposure. Prematurely uncovering such secrets can retraumatize rather than heal. Masud Khan (1974) warned that psychoanalysis must respect the patient's right to privacy, distinguishing between defensive concealment that hampers development and a necessary support for self-cohesion.

Furthermore, analysts must cultivate reverie and embodied listening. Much of the secret life of the patient is conveyed nonverbally: through bodily gestures, tone of voice, rhythms of engagement and withdrawal. Attending to these modes of communication requires the analyst to be in touch with their own bodily and affective responses, their own secret resonances. Sometimes the patient's secret is first "spoken" in the analyst's countertransference.

The timing of interpretations is crucial. Interpretations that reveal the analyst's superior knowledge too early can collapse the patient's protective structures and lead to feelings of exposure or violation. Analytic work involves waiting with the patient's hiddenness, allowing meanings to ripen and be discovered together rather than imposed. Here, a clinical example may be helpful: A young man entered therapy ostensibly for anxiety. Over time, it became clear through subtle bodily cues—nervous foot tapping when discussing intimacy, tightened shoulders when speaking about family—that an important secret lay hidden. Rather than confronting the patient with interpretations about potential sexual or familial secrets, the analyst allowed the bodily signs to be noticed, held, and eventually mirrored back empathically. Months later, the patient disclosed a deeply buried experience of sexual trauma that he had never told anyone, an experience surrounded by shame, confusion, and dissociation. The respectful waiting—trusting the secret riverbeds of the body and the analytic field—allowed a disclosure that could be metabolized.

Analysts must remain attuned to the co-construction of secrecy in the analytic relationship itself. Patients may enact old patterns of secrecy with the analyst, but analysts may also unconsciously collude with these patterns—through avoidance, rescue fantasies, or over-curiosity. Supervision and ongoing self-analysis are vital to detect when the analyst is becoming a participant in the maintenance or rupture of the secret space.

Working with secrecy psychoanalytically demands a deep ethical sensitivity. It is not a matter of "exposing" the patient's hidden truths but of accompanying them along the winding, unseen riverbeds of their psychic life—bearing witness, offering containment, and trusting that the patient will reveal what needs to be revealed in their own time and in their own way.

Future Directions

Often approached in psychoanalytic thought as a defensive maneuver or pathological symptom, secrecy constitutes a profound and inevitable dimension of subjectivity. From Freud's vault of the unconscious, Ferenczi's "confusion of tongues," to Klein's internal phantasies; from Fairbairn's and Guntrip's secret inner worlds to Winnicott's reverent "unfound self" and Bollas's (1987) "unthought known," it appears not as an aberration but as a feature of psychic life.

Integration of psychoanalytic insights with existential and philosophical perspectives—Buber's dialogic space, Levinas's ethics of alterity, Heidegger's concealment of Being—reveals that secrecy is not the enemy of relationality but its condition. To encounter the Other ethically is not to know everything, but to accompany what remains hidden. These intersections deepen our view of secrecy as a form of knowing that precedes telling.

Psychoanalytic therapy, in this light, becomes not the extraction of secrets but a practice of listening to the psychic landscape they leave behind. It is a negotiation of what must be said and what must be protected, what seeks light and what needs shadow. Sometimes, the secret may be gradually spoken; sometimes, it must be allowed to exist in the shared silence between analyst and patient. Rather than viewing secrets as obstacles, we might see them as riverbeds guiding the flow of psychic life. Our task is not to drain them dry, but to walk alongside them with care.

This inquiry opens more doors than it closes; a few of its limitations may guide future exploration.

First, this analysis has largely drawn upon psychoanalytic theories rooted in Western thought. Cross-cultural perspectives on secrecy—how different societies conceptualize private life, communal boundaries, and the ethics of disclosure—remain underexplored. Future research might integrate anthropological and sociocultural studies to understand secrecy's varied manifestations across diverse contexts.

Furthermore, while the provided clinical vignettes illustrate broad dynamics, they cannot capture the full complexity of long-term analytic work. More detailed process accounts, following secrecy's unfolding across years of treatment, would offer richer insights into its clinical negotiation. The relationship between secrecy and developmental trauma, particularly complex and cumulative trauma, warrants elaboration. How early experiences of betrayal, neglect, or boundary violation influence the construction of secret selves remains an area ripe for deeper integration with contemporary trauma theory and attachment research. Finally, the philosophical engagement offers a number of other pathways for the nuanced psychoanalytic conceptions of what remains hidden in human life.

Future psychoanalytic work could benefit from explicitly linking secrecy to the research on implicit memory, somatic markers, and "unformulated experience" (Solms & Turnbull, 2002; Stern, 2003). Such interdisciplinary bridges could illuminate how secrets live not only in language but in neural and bodily systems.

A richer understanding of secrecy also offers clinical hope. Recognizing the hidden life of the patient may be the very terrain where true transformation begins.

2 Defenses against Aliveness

Safety, Shame, and the Inhibition of Contact

This chapter examines how psychic defenses not only protect against pain or trauma, but also against vitality itself. Across a range of clinical and theoretical contexts, it considers how aliveness can become unbearable—too unregulated, too demanding, too revealing—and is thus disavowed, stylized, or withheld. Drawing on object relations, affect theory, and contemporary relational thought, the chapter traces multiple defensive structures: inhibition, splitting, manic performance, seductive absence, and ghosted vitality. Clinical vignettes illustrate how each form of defense structures time, relation, and the analyst's countertransference. Rather than frame aliveness as an obvious good, the chapter attends to its ambivalence—its psychic cost and its haunting return. It closes by reflecting on the analyst's role not as a restorer of lost feeling, but as a witness to its deferred traces.

The Threat of Aliveness

Some patients do not fear death so much as they fear vitality. Aliveness—emotional, relational, erotic—is too unstable to tolerate. It implies movement, desire, and the risk of contact. Where death can be imagined as stillness or cessation, aliveness carries the unbearable possibility of surprise. It asks something of the self. It calls for participation. And in the presence of early or repeated misattunement, this call can feel less like an invitation and more like a trap.

Aliveness, in this chapter, refers not simply to exuberance or animation, but to the psychic condition in which the self is allowed to feel, to reach, to respond. It is Winnicott's spontaneous gesture, Loewald's symbolic rhythm, and Panksepp's affective system seeking resonance. Yet for some patients, the cost of this resonance is too high. Vitality is associated with exposure; to be moved is to be open to violation. The analytic task, then, is not to coax the patient into liveliness, but to understand how and why that liveliness has been bracketed, stalled, or defended against.

Many of the patients we call "flat," "performative," or "resistant" are not defending against insight or contact itself, but against the dangerous sequelae of aliveness. They are managing affect at the level of metabolic threshold.

DOI: 10.4324/9781003715283-4

As Jaak Panksepp's work on affective neuroscience suggests, shame—along with its close neighbors panic and grief—is a fundamental organizing affect. It is not simply a social feeling but a mammalian signal: something has gone wrong in the space between. Shame is often read as withdrawal or collapse, but underneath, it is about unbearable exposure. The organism that expects connection and receives misattunement must find a way to limit further harm. One of the most efficient ways to do so is to inhibit aliveness altogether.

Judith Butler has written that vulnerability is not merely a condition of injury but a condition of being addressable. To be alive in the presence of another is to be available for response. In early developmental failures, this availability may be met not with recognition but with intrusion, neglect, or shame. The child learns, sometimes with exquisite precision, how to remain within relational proximity while muting the very signals that would call for mutuality. This is the root of many false self structures—not grand performance, but a quiet wariness around being too real, too soon.

Jessica Benjamin offers a different angle on the same phenomenon. In her language, recognition is a mutual act, one in which each subject affirms the other as separate and alive. But where recognition fails, especially early and often, the self may learn to organize around control rather than mutuality. Aliveness becomes risky because it invites unpredictability, the other's response, and the breakdown of symmetry. Patients who have not internalized the possibility of shared affect may experience liveliness not as expansion but as rupture. In such cases, the most self-protective act is to dampen affect, to manage vitality like a dangerous current.

Clinically, these defenses manifest in subtle and often misinterpreted ways. Some patients arrive with flat tone, constrained gesture, and a narrative style that never quite lets you in. Others may seem lively, even charismatic, but the energy is defensive—performative, evasive, calibrated to keep something unspoken from breaking through. In both cases, the analytic pair may find themselves caught in a paradox: aliveness is both what the patient longs for and what they cannot tolerate. The work must proceed not by calling forth more spontaneity, but by attending to the very structure that inhibits it, not as pathology, but as wisdom.

This chapter explores how patients defend against aliveness—not as a rejection of life, but as a compromise with what life has required them to survive. It is not a chapter about vitality in its exuberant forms, but about its retreat. Through clinical vignettes and theoretical elaboration, we will trace how inhibition functions not as absence, but as structure. Not as a failure, but as a symbolic delay. And we will explore how the analyst's presence—embodied, rhythmic, and restrained—may offer not liberation, but co-regulation. A way of being with what has been too alive to bear.

Withholding and the Fear of Being Seen

She arrived each week with a quiet precision that was difficult to name but impossible to miss. Her clothing was tasteful and unremarkable; her expressions were controlled, and her stories were coherent. She never canceled. She rarely cried. And yet, despite the surface smoothness of our work, I often left the session feeling like I hadn't really met her. She was not evasive. She was present. But it was a presence without contact, a proximity without mutuality. I could hear her words, but I couldn't feel their source.

At first, I mistook this restraint for stability. She described her week, shared her thoughts, and responded to interpretations with polite interest. There was no apparent resistance, no dramatic enactments, no high-stakes transference. But over time, I began to realize that what was absent was not material, but vitality. Her sessions moved forward, but did not deepen. They were organized around a kind of affective starvation that did not cry out, but settled in.

In one session, she described a moment of joy she'd had at a family gathering—a niece's laugh, a shared look, a trace of levity. "It was nice," she said, then quickly moved on. I paused, gently returning to the moment. "What did it feel like to laugh with her like that?" She looked at me blankly for a beat, then said, "I don't know. It wasn't a big deal." But something flickered—a break in rhythm, a loss of her usual smoothness. She looked down. "I guess it's hard to talk about that stuff."

Later, she would say: "It's embarrassing to feel too much." Not because she distrusted emotion per se, but because something in her early life had taught her that feelings were not welcome in the room. Her father was stern, her mother often overwhelmed. "They liked me best when I was quiet. Good. Not needy." Emotional self-expression was not punished directly, but subtly starved. She was not met, only tolerated.

What emerged in our work was not dramatic trauma, but a kind of quiet deprivation—a misattunement that structured her psyche around inhibition. To express liveliness, joy, or even sadness had become a kind of relational exposure she could not afford. Her defenses were not armored; they were almost moral. She did not feel she was hiding. She felt she was behaving.

Over time, her compliance began to function as a kind of defense mechanism, serving as a kind of transference shield. I would interpret, and she would agree. I would empathize, and she would nod. But the room remained thin. The shame beneath her withholding was rarely named directly, but it hung between us like static. It was not shame about specific actions or desires, but about being visible at all. The shame of being seen wanting. The shame of being seen as needing.

When she did begin to thaw, it was not through catharsis, but through micro-movements—a longer pause, a sigh she didn't retract, a story that ended without resolution. These were small acts of self-disclosure that felt almost dangerous to her. Not because she feared judgment, but because she feared becoming real in the presence of another.

At one point, after I gently observed her tendency to minimize pleasure, she asked, "Is it bad that I don't feel more?" The question wasn't defensive; it was genuinely curious. I said, "I don't think it's bad. I think it's protective." She looked at me and nodded, slowly. "Yeah. I guess it never felt safe to enjoy something too much." The statement was quiet, but it carried an emotional weight that lingered for weeks.

This patient was not resisting connection. She was surviving it. Her withholding was not avoidance, but attunement—to a world that had offered more scrutiny than recognition. Her inhibition of aliveness was not an absence of feeling, but a learned restraint against the unbearable risk of contact.

What Must Be Hidden: Shame, Love, and the Moral Defense

The affect that most needed to be repressed, Fairbairn observed, was not rage or aggression—but love. For the child confronted with unresponsive, misattuned, or punitive caregivers, the experience of loving becomes unbearable. Not because love is absent, but because it is met with failure, distortion, or emptiness. In such conditions, loving becomes dangerous. It exposes the self to psychic injury. And in response, the child does not cease to love—they cease to express it. They become quiet, composed, and withheld. The inhibition of aliveness is not a renunciation of life, but a compromise formation—a strategy to preserve coherence under threat.

The clinical presentation that results is often misread as emptiness. But it is not an absence—it is a structure. Inhibition of affect becomes a form of containment, a symbolic scaffolding to hold something far more volatile: the risk of tenderness, the terror of exposure, the catastrophe of being unmet. Fairbairn's formulation of the **moral defense** adds another layer. The child internalizes the failure of the object as their own ethical inadequacy. "If I am unmet, it must be because I am bad." Over time, this becomes a foundational structure of identity. Affect is not just repressed; it is framed as wrong. To feel is to err. To desire is to risk rupture. The false self that emerges is not a mask—it is a **moral solution** to an impossible relational field.

This was true of the patient described in the previous section. Her inhibition was not blankness but vigilance, shaped by early lessons in how not to disturb others. Her emotional restraint had the texture of goodness. Her compliance carried an ethical weight. In her family, wanting was to be a burden. To enjoy was to stand out. Her vitality—when it flickered—seemed to frighten her. It was not just shameful. It was forbidden.

Melanie Klein offers another lens here. In *Notes on Some Schizoid Mechanisms* (1946), she describes how the psyche defends itself against fragmentation through **splitting**—dividing the good and bad parts of self and object to maintain coherence. In the face of overwhelming ambivalence, the infant splits what cannot yet be integrated. Love and hate cannot coexist safely. Desire and danger collapse into one another. For such patients, aliveness becomes psychically unmanageable not because it is inherently too much, but because it cannot be held in integrated form. The self must divide in order to survive.

Yet it is important to note—and the book will return to this in *The Original Paradox*—that **splitting is not inherently pathological**. It is the **earliest form**

of psychic organization, the first gesture by which the subject begins to differentiate, to locate itself in relation to experience. In early life, and often again under trauma, splitting offers a rudimentary architecture for self-preservation. It is both a division and a beginning. The danger arises not from the fact of splitting, but from its rigidity: when the split becomes fixed, unyielding, incapable of metabolizing contradiction or generating symbolic transformation.

In this light, **psychic disintegration** is not merely a breakdown of ego functioning or a loss of cognitive control. It is a collapse of the self's symbolic coherence: the loss of sequence, containment, rhythm, and recognizability. Affective states flood the system without modulation. Thought cannot follow feeling. The body may register everything—shame, panic, dread—without the psyche being able to narrate it. In Loewald's terms, it is a failure of symbolization; in Klein's terms, it is the unbinding of experience into raw, persecutory fragments. The dread is not only that one will feel too much, but that one will **cease to exist as a subject** in time.

Guntrip extends this insight through his articulation of **annihilation anxiety**—a pre-symbolic terror that one's subjective selfhood may vanish in the face of relational intensity. The schizoid patient does not merely withdraw from contact; they retreat into a sealed interiority to preserve a self that feels too fragile to survive a relationship. Love is not simply longed for and feared. It is experienced as a consuming force, a fire that could incinerate the thin, papered walls of the self. To remain intact, the patient must remain hidden. Their inhibition becomes a sanctuary.

One such patient, not unlike the first but more imaginative in his detachment, often spoke with expressive verbal fluidity. He described dreamlike internal scenes, distant memories, and philosophical musings with fluency and even flair. And yet, week after week, he left no affective trace. His words evoked affect, but he did not seem to feel it. He often described feelings as though they belonged to someone else. "I imagine I was quite lonely," he once said of his childhood. "It must have been difficult." The statement was articulate, but hollow. I noticed that my own experience of the session mirrored his—lucid, articulate, and affectively vacated.

At times, I found myself admiring his verbal elegance, even as I felt gently anesthetized in the room. Later, I realized that he was not avoiding me. He was avoiding himself. The vitality he preserved was stored in language, symbol, and private myth—but it could not yet enter the relational field. Like many schizoid patients, he had developed a rich inner life that served as both refuge and defense. The analytic space was tolerated, but rarely inhabited. He was not absent. He was **elsewhere**.

Klein's notion of **projective identification** helps clarify what happens here: affective states that cannot be owned are lodged in the analyst. With this patient, I felt a paradoxical pressure to remain clear-headed and articulate—disavowing my own emotional complexity to match the neutrality of the field. I began to feel like an echo chamber, not a participant. What he disowned, I absorbed. This was not resistance. It was field survival.

In such cases, **envy** may also operate quietly. Klein suggests that the patient may unconsciously attack their own emerging pleasure or spontaneity, which is experienced as too risky, too hopeful, or too aligned with lost or dangerous objects. To feel joy might be to betray the depressive mother, to feel spontaneity might be to abandon the withdrawn father. These identifications are often unconscious, but their impact is pervasive. The self remains withheld not only from fear, but from **loyalty**—to the broken world that shaped it.

This is what makes these defenses so difficult to approach. They do not feel like symptoms. They feel like ethics, like safety, like wisdom. The patient is not simply defending against liveliness. They are defending against longing, shame, and the internal collapse that would follow unmet need. They are defending against disintegration. Against the terror of needing someone who cannot hold them. Against the risk of a self that might emerge too vividly, only to vanish again.

These defenses must be honored as achievements. But they also mark a threshold. For the patient organized around inhibition, the question is not "Can I feel?" but "Is it survivable to be seen?" As we move toward the schizoid compromise in the next section, we carry forward this understanding: that what looks like withdrawal is often a final defense against psychic extinction. And that the analyst's task is not to pierce it, but to dwell near it long enough that something else might begin to stir.

The Schizoid Compromise

Not all who inhibit aliveness are schizoid. But all who inhibit aliveness, in some sense, contain within them a schizoid compromise: a private refusal of relational danger, a carefully walled-off center around which the rest of psychic life is built. While classically understood as a personality organization marked by detachment and inner withdrawal, the schizoid structure can also be viewed more fundamentally—as a symbolic strategy: an internal contract that trades mutuality for survivability. To touch the other, it assumes, is to risk annihilation.

This structure is not limited to schizoid character per se. Beneath the surface of many personality configurations lies a hidden nucleus—a schizoid seed, formed when the self discovers, early and without language, that being fully present in the field of the other is unbearable. The self doesn't disappear; it retreats. It doesn't cease to feel; it buries affect in private chambers of fantasy, ritual, intellect, or silence. Over time, this retreat becomes its own reality, defended not only against others but against the self's own longing. The schizoid seed survives by organizing the conditions under which aliveness is no longer allowed to circulate.

This seed is universal. It is present in the manic patient who discharges energy into hypervitality to avoid stillness. It is present in the narcissistic patient who constructs a dazzling, controlling surface to avoid the chaos of being seen unscripted. It is present in the depressive patient who has relinquished joy in unconscious loyalty to a fragile, depleted parent. In each case, the personality style is a choreography around a kernel of terror—that to show up fully, emotionally, is to be pierced or obliterated. The self is not resisting relationship. It is resisting collapse.

What makes this seed so difficult to detect is that it does not always manifest in the absence. Sometimes it is flamboyant, intellectual, performative, or highly verbal. But what remains constant is the protective closure—the refusal to let affect circulate freely in the relational field. What is defended against is not feeling per se, but the symbolic risk of mutuality: the unknown, the unscripted, the metabolically alive.

Freud's concept of repetition compulsion offered a foundational account of how the psyche relives what it cannot symbolize. In *Beyond the Pleasure Principle*, he observed that trauma often returns not as memory, but as re-enactment—a circular return of the unassimilated. But what we encounter in the schizoid compromise is not simply repetition. It is recursion—a looping structure that lacks awareness of itself as a loop. Where repetition seeks mastery, recursion seeks safety. There is no active redramatization; only the indistinction between past and present remains. The patient doesn't believe they are re-enacting anything. They believe they are being careful, thoughtful, moral, and restrained. The danger is not in the memory; it is in the structure of time itself.

The schizoid seed bends temporality into a Möbius strip: a surface with one continuous side, no entry point, and no exit. The past does not return. It simply never ends. What feels like the present is often the past, folded inward, mistaken for now. Experience becomes recursive rather than transformative. The self is not closed to contact—it is unaware that contact is even missing.

One patient, a writer in his thirties, illustrated this beautifully. His sessions were dense, layered, and intellectually brilliant. He would describe scenes of his life with intricate nuance, often noting the ironies or mythic resonances of events. He spoke of emotion often—but from outside it. "It's strange," he said once. "I can describe my sadness, but I don't think I've ever actually felt it." His affect was neither flat nor exaggerated. It was distilled—converted into a metaphor before it could be metabolized in the room. I found myself moved by his words, but unanchored. I realized I was grieving for a sadness I could feel more than he could. And that, perhaps, was his unconscious arrangement.

As our work deepened, it became clear that he had internalized a world in which knowing had replaced feeling. He had learned to survive through narrative curation—through being the one who interprets, not the one who feels. His inner life was alive, even beautiful, but it could not be entered by the analytic field. The room was structured to keep mutual affect at bay, not through hostility, but through subtle dislocation. The Möbius structure was intact: what felt immediate was always already encoded.

The analyst's countertransference in such work is often muted, paradoxical. One may feel intellectually engaged but emotionally vacated, like a guest in a perfectly curated museum with no entry to the artist's studio. The desire to "wake" the patient can be strong—but must be resisted. The structure was not built to deceive. It was built to hold. And it will not be softened through pressure. The analyst's task is to dwell near the sealed structure, to become a temporal companion rather than an interpreter of absence.

But the schizoid seed is not exclusive to the inward-turning. It wears many disguises.

The manic patient often escapes the Möbius loop not by collapsing it but by fleeing it altogether—living in temporal excess. Every moment is forward-driven, every silence interrupted by speech, gesture, stimulation. Yet the undercurrent is the same: stillness is unendurable. To pause might invite collapse. The manic flight is not vitality—it is evasion. The inner void is not healed; it is outrun.

The narcissistic patient may appear confident, present, and even emotionally attuned—until spontaneity arises. The moment becomes unscripted, and a subtle chill enters the field. Their performance of authenticity is precise, but privately structured to disavow vulnerability. Praise is metabolized. Intimacy is destabilizing. Beneath the surface charm, the schizoid seed curls tightly around a singular fear: if I am known, I will be destroyed.

The depressive patient, by contrast, may feel the loss of aliveness explicitly. But it is often structured as a sacrifice rather than an absence—a giving-up of vitality in the service of preserving the object. The seed here is relational loyalty. Joy becomes dangerous because it risks disturbing the parent's pain. In such patients, the split is not between self and other, but between inner permission and outer mourning.

In all of these structures, the schizoid seed loops temporality into the same recursive fold. What Bion described as an "attack on linking" becomes not just a disruption of thought, but a refusal of symbolic time. Loewald helps us here: symbolization, for him, is the transformation of raw experience into temporally structured psychic life. When symbolization fails, experience cannot be metabolized. It cannot become past. It cannot move. The self is not traumatized by events. It is traumatized by its inability to process them in time. The patient does not repeat because they remember. They repeat because they cannot think of anything else to do.

This is where Freud's theory meets its recursive mirror. Repetition compulsion assumes a subject who re-enacts. However, in the schizoid compromise, the structure itself repeats. The subject is enclosed inside the Möbius loop, where repetition has lost its symbolic intent. It is not mastery that is being sought. It is containment without contact.

This brings us to a wider reflection: that Freudian, neo-Freudian, and object relational theories each refract some facet of this phenomenon. Freud located repetition in the return of the repressed. Sullivan emphasized interpersonal safety and the co-construction of defensive patterns. Klein, Fairbairn, and Guntrip revealed how internal objects are stabilized through splitting, idealization, and withdrawal. But none of these traditions fully maps the recursive time structure of the schizoid compromise. And yet, together, they sketch a topology: a psychic architecture where contact threatens coherence, and survival is structured as detachment. These theoretical lenses—Freudian, interpersonal, object-relational—each catch a shard of lived experience. Each helps us see the defensive fold. But none alone captures the Möbius curvature of defended life. The schizoid seed sits behind all of them, organizing what can be symbolized and what must be looped.

In this light, the analytic task shifts. We do not interpret resistance as obstruction. We recognize it as continuity—the very fabric of the patient's psychic coherence. We do not seek to extract the real self from behind the false one. We accompany the recursion. We let the Möbius strip unfold in our presence, not to break it, but to mark it with time.

Sometimes, this occurs through a moment of silence that the patient does not rush to fill. Sometimes through an image, a sigh, a forgotten word. These are not breakthroughs. They are deviations in the loop—evidence that something new has touched the structure, even if only briefly.

As we move toward the final sections of this chapter, we begin to see that transformation does not mean dismantling the compromise. It means accompanying it until it begins to shift. Not quickly, and not completely. But enough that the loop bends toward symbolization. Enough that the self may come to feel not only contained—but met.

Performance as Defense: The Panic of Being Known

Not all inhibition takes the form of quiet. Some forms of inhibition are loud, bright, even magnetic. Patients organized around performance often appear lively, expressive, articulate—even seductive. But beneath the fluency lies a deeper structure: not aliveness, but panic. For these patients, performance becomes a defense not only against psychic collapse, but against the risk of being seen without choreography.

This is a different flavor of false self than we've seen in the previous sections. The patient is not restrained or withdrawn. They are animated. They tell vivid stories, express strong feelings, and appear deeply engaged in the analytic process. But something is missing. Their self-expression, while compelling, does not feel metabolized. The analytic field is full of words but strangely devoid of contact. The performance is not insincere—it is overdetermined. It is a way of filling the space so that nothing unexpected can enter.

One patient, a mid-career creative professional, illustrated this dynamic with striking clarity. From the first session, she was warm, articulate, and emotionally literate. She reflected easily on her childhood, named her fears and longings with apparent transparency, and often spoke of her desire for "real connection." Her stories were rich with texture, irony, and pathos. I found myself admiring her self-awareness, laughing at her jokes, and moved by her insights. And yet, after several months, I began to notice a paradoxical fatigue. I was emotionally stirred, but never quite included. Something in me remained just outside the scene.

Her narrative was exquisitely timed—gestures, intonations, confessions arriving with theatrical precision. Moments of silence were rare, and when they came, she filled them quickly with apology or humor. If I offered an interpretation that didn't land smoothly, she pivoted deftly, steering us back into familiar terrain. She had an uncanny ability to produce resonance, but not to inhabit it. Her affect was expressive but not porous. She performed rather than exposing it.

Over time, a pattern became clear. The patient's vitality was real—but it was staged. Behind the spontaneity was an invisible script. Her relational field was saturated with anticipation of how I might respond, what I might want, where the conversation might go. What looked like openness was, in fact, a subtle form of control. Not to dominate me, but to prevent the unknown from entering the space. Her greatest fear was not rejection. It was interruption—being caught off guard, unrehearsed, unready.

Winnicott's concept of the false self is helpful here, particularly his distinction between the compliant false self and the creative true self. While later chapters will explore the false self more fully—not as mere pathology, but as a complex, time-bound adaptation—this vignette offers a window into one of its livelier forms. The patient was not compliant in the conventional sense. She did not suppress her personality or tone down her emotions. But she lived in an anticipatory posture—constantly attuned to what might be expected of her, what might be pleasing, what might ensure relational coherence. Her false self was not silent. It was dazzling. It protected her from collapse not through withdrawal, but through a flood of expressiveness. Winnicott notes that when the false self takes over entirely, it may function "in ways that make it impossible for the true self to find external reality to which to relate." In this case, the performance did not suppress the true self—it shielded it so thoroughly that even the patient could not feel when it was absent.

This dynamic also evokes Bollas's notion of the "unthought known"—those early, pre-verbal experiences that shape psychic structure without becoming symbolized. For this patient, something about stillness, surprise, or rupture was associated with danger. If she was not in control of the tempo, the rhythm, or the emotional arc, something in her body registered panic. She did not know why—only that spontaneity felt like freefall. Her charm was not simply social. It was regulatory.

My own countertransference mirrored this logic. I felt impressed, appreciative, even entertained—but never needed. I began to question whether I mattered to her at all. But slowly, I realized this was not a dismissal. It was a defense. If I were too central, too real, too unpredictable, I might interrupt the choreography—and with it, her psychic equilibrium. I wasn't being excluded. I was being kept in a role: an audience, not a partner.

Bion's theory of contact barriers helps us understand what was occurring at a deeper level. For Bion, the psyche must have a permeable membrane that allows for the digestion of emotional experience—what he calls alpha-function. In this case, the patient's membrane was dense with anticipatory material. Feelings were converted into action, reflection, or disclosure before they could be metabolized. The analytic container was bypassed. Performance ensured that nothing lingered long enough to become disruptive.

This dynamic is not confined to the high-functioning, relationally sophisticated patient. The defensive use of performance spans structures. In some, it takes a manic form—full of charisma, restlessness, and improvisational energy. In others, it arrives in hysteric registers: affectively vivid, emotionally charged, and entangled in the gaze of the other.

A young man in his 20s illustrated this manic variation. He arrived at each session overflowing with narrative. Dreams, insights, heartbreaks, political analysis, childhood memories, and jokes. His mind was agile, his language kinetic. Sessions moved fast. I often left feeling intoxicated by his liveliness—and then abruptly emptied. Something wasn't settling. Over time, it became clear that his brilliance was a form of dissociation, not from trauma per se, but from unstructured presence. He could not tolerate the stillness of mutual regard. If I paused too long, his speech accelerated. If I commented on something emotional, he changed the subject. If I made a mistake, he forgave it too quickly. He was never quite in the moment because being in the moment meant losing his footing. Charm was a defense against psychic gravity.

In these patients, the performance is not cynical or manipulative. It is sacralized. It has become a life raft. Their survival has depended on evoking a response without ever being in it. The gaze of the other is necessary, but unbearable. They seek recognition that doesn't arrive too soon, too sharp, too naked. And when it does, they recoil—not from contempt, but from the terror of contact they can't control.

For the analyst, this creates a unique challenge. We are moved, engaged, even enchanted—but often subtly disoriented. Our attention is drawn toward the narrative and away from the field. If we are not careful, we begin to enact the very structure we are meant to witness. We become reliable consumers of the performance rather than co-participants in its gradual softening.

In these cases, interpretation is rarely useful in the conventional sense. What is required is not confrontation, but containment. The analyst must become a rhythmic partner, not a dramaturg. Our task is to help metabolize what was never permitted to unfold—to slow the choreography until it begins to shimmer and strain.

Sometimes, this means allowing the loop to run until it exhausts itself. Other times, it means gently disturbing the rhythm—not with accusation, but with curiosity. "I notice you moved quickly past that moment," one might say. Or: "Something in the room felt different when you looked away—did you feel it too?" These interventions are not interpretive in and of themselves. They are temporal nudges—small invitations to notice that the dance has a tempo and that someone else is here.

Winnicott wrote that the false self protects the true self from impingement until conditions are right for emergence. But he also warned that when the false self becomes a full-time caretaker, the true self risks atrophy. Later chapters will return to this paradox in detail—how the false self, though adaptive, may ultimately obscure the self it was meant to protect. Here, we see the beginnings of that risk. The patient has built an aesthetic of presence so polished that actual presence becomes unbearable. What was once a creative adaptation now functions as a recursive trap. The self becomes legible only in performance and unlivable in its absence.

The performance is not just defensive—it is a rescue fantasy. If I stay animated, I won't be dropped. If I keep you laughing, you won't notice I'm scared. If I perform a connection, I won't be asked to feel it. Over time, the fantasy hardens into identity. And yet, something in the patient still longs to be met—not as a performer, but as a person. It is this longing that the analyst must protect, even when the patient seems intent on obscuring it.

In supervision, I once remarked on a patient like this, "He's so compelling I forget to feel." That sentence stayed with me. The work, I realized, was not to see through the performance, but to feel with it—to let it affect me, but not consume the field. The analyst must become a partner in containment, a witness to the pacing, and a co-architect of a more livable rhythm.

When this goes well, something shifts. Not all at once. Not dramatically. But slowly, the patient begins to pause. Their gestures lose their rehearsed shine. A sentence stumbles. A joke falls flat—and is not rescued. These are not failures. They are signs of a new psychic tempo. The performance no longer needs to do all the work.

In one session with the original patient described above, she spoke of a recent interaction that had left her feeling unseen. She described it beautifully, employing metaphors and emotionally charged language. I nodded. Then, unexpectedly, she stopped mid-sentence. "Wait," she said, "I think I'm doing it again. I'm narrating instead of feeling." She looked down, took a breath, and said, "Actually, I was devastated. And I still kind of am." The room went quiet. She didn't try to fix it. And I didn't try to interpret it. We just sat there.

In that moment, the performance loosened. Not because she gave it up, but because she let me join her behind it.

The Erotics of Withdrawal: When Aliveness Must Be Refused

Not all defenses against aliveness are retreats into isolation. Some are invitations cloaked in refusal. There are patients for whom withholding is not just protection from overwhelm, but a mode of relational control—a carefully curated absence that exerts force. These patients do not withdraw to disappear. They withdraw to become *felt*. The retreat is not an escape from contact but a reconfiguration of it: power through distance, erotic charge through absence, affective regulation through a refusal to arrive.

This is not the schizoid compromise explored earlier, where withdrawal defends against annihilation through structural dissociation. Here, withdrawal is saturated with agency. The patient may be charming, compelling, even magnetic, but always just out of reach. Their vitality is not collapsed; it is withheld. Something is being held back—not because it cannot be given, but because its withholding is the point.

One patient, a reserved but elegant man in his forties, brought this dynamic into focus. He arrived promptly each week, well-groomed, engaged, and emotionally articulate—but with a strange sense of distance that felt choreographed. He would share stories from his life, often painful or intimate in content, but told with a stylized remove. "I know this is sad," he would say, with a half-smile, "but I've gotten used to it." His affect was never quite absent, but always buffered—textured by self-awareness, wry intelligence, and aesthetic control.

Over time, I began to feel a subtle yet persistent ache in our sessions. Not frustration, exactly—more like yearning. I wanted him to arrive emotionally. I wanted to feel him in the room in a way that matched the material. But the very sense of incompleteness began to feel like his unconscious offering. He never refused connection directly; he simply made it rare. His presence became something I was subtly waiting for. And he seemed to know it.

This is the erotic economy of withdrawal. Presence becomes a scarce resource, and its scarcity creates gravity. The patient is not seducing in the classical sense. But their refusal to be fully present produces desire—in the analyst, in others, in themselves. Something about being withheld becomes metabolically charged. They control not by dominance, but by deferring mutuality just enough to generate longing.

Freud's theory of masochism offers one entry into this terrain. In his 1924 paper on "The Economic Problem of Masochism," Freud describes how passivity may become a route to mastery. The masochist organizes suffering as a means of psychic control—turning the object's power into a staged drama where pain becomes choice. In this frame, withdrawal may not be feared. It may be a command. The patient withholds not because they cannot connect, but because not connecting is how they remain intact. There is pleasure in the refusal. Not sadism, necessarily, but structure. Affect is managed by keeping the other just far enough away.

Fairbairn's theory of internal object relations adds another layer. For Fairbairn, the child internalizes rejecting or unresponsive objects not merely as painful, but as morally binding. The ego becomes split, with one part identified with the withholding object and another with the denied, degraded self. This creates a tragic loyalty: to repeat the experience of being unmet as a way of preserving the internal structure of early attachment. In the adult patient, this may manifest as a stylized withdrawal that both protects and punishes. The analyst is cast as the one who must yearn and wait, just as the patient once did. Only now is the patient in control.

In such cases, the withdrawal becomes a performance of power—not aggressive, but precise. The patient does not dominate the analyst. They organize the rhythm. They decide when intimacy becomes possible. They signal openness, then turn subtly away. The analyst is drawn in, then pauses.

The countertransference is often erotic, but not because the patient is overtly seductive. Rather, it is the staged incompleteness that arouses. The room fills with tension, not because anything is happening, but because something isn't.

As our work deepened, the patient's style of absence became more pronounced. If I asked how he felt in the moment, he would smile slightly, then respond with a memory. If I named something emotional, he would agree warmly but leave it untouched. One day, after I shared a particularly resonant reflection, he said simply, "That's lovely," and then changed the subject. I realized then that even my best attunement was being curated into distance. He wanted to be witnessed—but not altered. He was not rejecting the connection. He was managing it.

My countertransference began to shift from gentle frustration to something more destabilizing. I noticed a subtle urgency rising in me. I wanted to break through the reserve, to elicit some sign that he needed me. I found myself rehearsing what I might say in the next session—how I could phrase things just right. I was no longer simply witnessing the withdrawal. I was *inside* it. The performance of absence had become our shared choreography. And I had been cast in the role of yearning.

This is part of what makes such dynamics so difficult to work with. The analyst is drawn not only into the patient's affective field but into their relational timing. We begin to wait, to hover, to anticipate. We are not pulled into grand enactments. We are slowed down to a tempo where our interventions feel too fast, our interpretations too presumptuous. The analyst's rhythm begins to reflect the withdrawal—controlled, delayed, reactive. And the patient remains slightly ahead of the moment, emotionally absent just long enough to avoid being reached.

Jessica Benjamin's writing on mutual recognition helps articulate the power at play here. For Benjamin, recognition requires both participants to be subjects—to risk being seen and to risk seeing. But in the dynamics of withdrawal, this mutuality is never quite allowed to form. The patient retains asymmetry as a mode of self-protection: they see us, but do not permit themselves to be seen. Or rather, they offer themselves to be seen in a way that neutralizes our gaze. They give just enough presence to suggest openness, but not enough to allow reciprocity. Recognition is invoked but not permitted.

This asymmetry can be seductive. The analyst feels close, but never quite essential. We become the witnesses to a beautifully maintained solitude, not its participant. And in that role, we are kept alive as objects—not abandoned, but also never quite real. The withdrawal preserves the patient's sense of agency by denying the analyst emotional leverage. If I do not fully arrive, you cannot fully affect me. If I do not reveal myself, I do not risk alteration. What appears as vulnerability is often calculated asymmetry, built to preserve self-definition.

Laplanche offers another register for understanding these dynamics. His concept of the enigmatic signifier—a message that is addressed to the subject but remains incompletely understood, untranslatable—resonates deeply with the eroticism of withdrawal. The patient's absence, in this sense, becomes a kind of signifier: not empty, but encrypted. The analyst receives the absence as meaningful, affectively charged, but cannot fully decode it. The patient's refusal to arrive becomes an event, a communication through what is not said. Their silences are saturated with unconscious messages that demand interpretation, but resist comprehension.

This is how withdrawal can become not a void, but a symbolic act. It shapes the field. It calls forth longing. It instills asymmetry. And it does so without any overt assertion of control. The patient is not manipulative; they are disciplined. Their absence is not a failure to show up. It is a way of scripting the encounter.

In such moments, the analyst's task is not to demand presence, but to bear its absence symbolically. We must hold the tension without resolving it. We must remain available without insisting. Sometimes, the most transformative act is not to ask the patient to come closer, but to recognize the meaning of their distance. To wait with them in the refusal—not as a strategy, but as a form of witnessing.

Eventually, the patient described a moment from childhood in which his mother, after a long silence, told him that he had always been "too much." He recounted it with the usual elegance. But then he paused. "I think I've spent my whole life trying to be just enough," he said, "which mostly means not needing anything." His voice faltered. For the first time, he didn't fill the space. I didn't speak. And something shifted. It wasn't catharsis. It was a pause that wasn't rehearsed. His presence was uncertain, but uncurated. The erotic withholding had cracked—not through confrontation, but through shared silence.

Withdrawal, when it functions as a defense, does not need to be dismantled. It needs to be accompanied. The analyst's role is not to restore aliveness, but to recognize its suspension as meaningful. To see that even in the absence of it, the patient is speaking. The refusal to be present is often the most reliable way they have ever had to remain intact. And paradoxically, it may be the only way they know how to reach.

Ghosts of Vitality: The Haunting of the Unexpressed

Defenses against aliveness do not always create silence. Sometimes, they create ghosts. Unexpressed vitality doesn't vanish; it lingers. It hovers at the edge of experience, never quite emerging, but never entirely gone. It haunts the psyche—not as the residue of trauma, but as the trace of potentiality: life that could have been lived, but wasn't.

This haunting is not just metaphorical. It takes form in mood, in repetition, in the strange feeling that something is missing even when nothing seems wrong. The analyst feels it in the atmosphere of the room. The patient may not seem acutely defensive, but the sessions are permeated with a kind of absence. Or sometimes, with an excess—an overly bright tone, a story that arrives too perfectly shaped, a laugh that feels unanchored. These are not just defenses against pain. They are signals of something unexpressed, trying to find its way back into time.

One patient, a woman in her early thirties, illustrated this dynamic through what I can only describe as a kind of beautiful melancholy. She was emotionally available, reflective, and full of aesthetic sensibility. She spoke often of her longings—not just for love, but for feeling "lit up," "moved," "sparked." Yet these desires were always framed in the past tense or projected into an indefinite future. Her present life, while functional and even rich in external ways, felt distant to her. "I know I'm supposed to be happy," she once said. "I have everything I thought I wanted. But there's this… fog. I'm here, but not quite."

Her affect was soft, sometimes wistful, occasionally animated—but rarely urgent. Even joy arrived gently, like a memory, not an event. It became clear that she was not simply inhibited or detached. She was haunted by a version of herself she had never fully become. Her vitality hadn't been lost. It had been deferred, displaced, and now lingered around the edges of her life like an echo.

In session, I often felt something just out of reach. She would share a memory or a fantasy, and I'd find myself holding my breath, waiting for something more to arrive. But it never did. The affective field was warm but muted. Her words were alive, but her presence was stylized. She could describe hunger without showing it. She could describe excitement without lighting up. The ghost of aliveness was everywhere—in her metaphors, her pace, her longing—but it never quite crossed the threshold into form.

Christopher Bollas's writing on the *crypt* and the fate of unlived life helps clarify this atmosphere. For Bollas, parts of the self that never found expression may be sequestered psychically, not in repression per se, but in a kind of aestheticized tomb. These parts do not erupt. They **seep**—into taste, into dream, into mood. The patient may appear reflective or refined, but something remains uncultivated. And the analyst feels it, not as a blockage, but as **aesthetic loss**: a presence that never quite arrives.

Michael Eigen offers a complementary frame. He writes of feeling states that saturate the analytic field not through content, but through **atmosphere**. Eigen speaks of haunted experience, not in the sense of ghost stories, but as a condition of being subtly surrounded by what one cannot fully feel. In these moments, the analytic task is not interpretation, but attunement to **ghosted aliveness**—affect that is no longer raw, but not yet alive.

With this patient, interpretation often felt too sharp. What she needed was space to let something unformed move. She did not fear collapse. She feared arriving too late for herself. Her life was not defended through inhibition or withdrawal. It was structured around **absence as a trace**—an ongoing elegy to parts of her psyche that had never been invited to participate in time.

Loewald helps us understand the temporal register of this phenomenon. For him, becoming is always delayed. The psyche does not unfold linearly, but in recursive gestures that return to the past in order to metabolize it forward. The patient's ghosted vitality was not just an artifact of missed experience—it was part of her ongoing structure of becoming. It was not what had failed to happen. It was what was still waiting for the right conditions to take form.

Not all ghosted vitality takes the form of absence. Sometimes it arrives as *too much*—a restless energy, a polished charisma, a force of presence that seems animated but uninhabited. These patients do not avoid affect; they evoke it. But their effect has no roots. It lights up the room and vanishes. They appear full of life, yet something remains unjoined. The liveliness feels displaced—as if their very animation is a strategy to avoid contact with something more elemental.

One patient, a man in his early forties, radiated presence. He was sharp, funny, emotionally expressive, even theatrically self-aware. He spoke freely about childhood pain, failed relationships, and existential fear—but always with a self-deprecating grace that kept me charmed. He performed vitally beautifully. But after each session, I noticed a strange heaviness in myself. It wasn't exhaustion, exactly. It was a feeling of loss—of having been moved, but not connected. Of having been near something alive, but never quite with it.

Over time, I came to recognize his charisma as a defense—not against depression or collapse, but against *gravity*. There was a refusal of depth beneath the sparkle, a refusal to slow down enough to feel. His liveliness was not false. It was curated. It was a means of *not stopping*. And what haunted the sessions was not what he couldn't say, but what kept trying to emerge between the performances: a grief so old it no longer had form. It had rhythm, but no name.

Antonio Damasio's work on somatic markers provides a helpful entry point here. He suggests that the body holds traces of affective experience even when it cannot be named—what he calls "somatic markers" that continue to shape perception, behavior, and mood. In patients like this, we might say that the body remembers what the psyche cannot symbolize. The emotional memory persists not in narrative, but in movement, tempo, and mood. The aliveness that was once disallowed has not disappeared—it has become misdirected energy, a performance of intensity in place of contact.

Michael Eigen's writing on "vital deadness" offers a parallel lens. He describes a condition in which the psyche becomes saturated with an absence that is too full to bear. Not numbness, but a deadening vibrancy—a state in which affect is present, even overwhelming, but unintegrated. In this state, the self organizes around the performance of aliveness to keep the true rhythm of feeling out of reach. The patient is not lifeless. They are overflowing with unfulfilled experiences, and their performance is both a communication and a shield.

In this patient, what needed to be witnessed was not the content of his disclosures, but their frequency and tempo. He was telling me everything, but never lingering. I slowed the sessions. I mirrored his cadence back to him. I let my silences stretch longer. At first, he laughed—"I'm making you work too hard, huh?" But gradually, the silences stopped being jokes. They became rooms. In one, he finally said, "I think I'm afraid of slowing down because

I don't know what would catch up to me." His voice cracked. The room quieted. He didn't move to fill the space. And neither did I.

Loewald helps us frame this as a movement from drive to symbol, from noise to voice. For him, the analyst does not interpret alone; the analyst lends time—making room for the patient's archaic, non-symbolized experiences to unfold in psychic sequence. Symbolization is not decoding. It is the restoration of rhythm. In this case, our task was not to expose the pain beneath the performance, but to allow the performance to soften, allowing something uncrafted to enter the field.

Ghosted vitality is not simply a symptom. It is a structure of mood. It hangs in the analytic space as a kind of pre-speech, a fugitive form of life. Its pressure is not always loud. Sometimes it is a sigh, a deflection, a glance that lingers too long. It is the moment in which nothing seems to happen, but everything is there.

These are the atmospheres that haunt defended patients—not because they are barren, but because they are overfull. The self carries the weight of unlived feeling, unclaimed desire, joy that was never shared. The haunting is not of what was, but of what never had a chance to be. And the analyst, if attuned, feels this not as absence, but as a presence that demands no interpretation—only recognition.

Analysis cannot restore the unlived. But it can make space for its residue. It can accompany the ghost—not to exorcise it, but to hear what it's still trying to say. Some parts of the psyche do not want to be revived. They want to be acknowledged. They want to know that someone finally stayed long enough to hear the life that never made it into words.

3 Erotic Submission

Aesthetic Stylization, Dissociation, and the Ethics of Presence

This paper explores erotic submission as a dissociative relational structure that enables affective survival after disrupted attachment and early trauma. Drawing on clinical material and relational theory, it considers how submission may serve as a regulatory choreography through which unbearable affect is managed without overwhelming the self. Rather than viewing submission as pathology or symptom, the analyst is positioned as a participant-witness to a carefully structured relational scene. Through disciplined attunement and embodied containment, the analyst enters a field where dissociated fragments of desire and recognition may begin to reorganize. The work does not aim to integrate prematurely but to hold the patient's relational aesthetic until it shifts on its own terms. In this stance, submission is neither valorized nor dismantled, but allowed to evolve. The analyst's ethical task is not to resolve contradiction, but to survive it—enabling the patient to risk presence, contact, and mutuality without psychic collapse.

Introduction and Theoretical Orientation

Erotic submission in the analytic setting is not always dramatic. It often arrives as a quiet rhythm—an arrangement of silences, deferments, and gestures that structure the patient's subjectivity as given-over, ambient, or displaced. The submission is not necessarily toward the analyst, nor even consciously toward another. Rather, it emerges as an aesthetic mode of self-organization: a choreography of dissociation through which relationality becomes possible.

This paper examines the phenomenon of erotic submission not as a perversion, symptom, or characterological defense, but as a dissociative and aesthetic form of psychic survival. Drawing from object relations theory, contemporary relational thought, and post-structural ethics, I propose that some patients live within eroticized structures of giving-over that allow them to remain in partial contact with affect, attachment, and selfhood. These are not enactments of masochism as Freud (1953b) imagined it, nor do they always resemble the dynamics described in more overt

DOI: 10.4324/9781003715283-5

presentations of sadomasochistic sexuality. Instead, they represent a quieter submission—one that forms when mutuality feels too dangerous, when recognition threatens psychic collapse, and when autonomy has been historically unlinked from safety.

The analyst in these treatments does not witness submission from outside. We are recruited into its structure—often as unknowing participants. We are idealized, disavowed, resisted, and longed for. We may find ourselves pulled into affective scenes that feel erotically charged, oddly flattened, or both. The patient may seem to offer themselves—psychically, emotionally, or erotically—but only within narrow parameters, often choreographed to avoid reciprocity. These dynamics are difficult to name and even harder to hold. But they are also clinically generative—offering a window into the patient's unconscious strategies for preserving relational coherence through stylized forms of dissociation.

As the work unfolds, the analyst is often left with an unspoken ethical task: to remain within the scene of submission without fully occupying the role offered. To feel into the erotically dissociated field without collapsing it through interpretation or retreat. The erotic, in these treatments, is often lodged in the aestheticized refusal of mutuality. It pulses through absence, not presence. To move too quickly toward integration—to insist on authenticity or clarity—is to violate the very structure that has allowed the patient to survive.

Stephen Mitchell (1988) writes that all desire is relational, even in its perversion or foreclosure. Jessica Benjamin (1995, 2004) extends this, arguing that mutual recognition is not always possible—and that failures of recognition are themselves constitutive of the relational field. For patients organized around erotic submission, recognition may be experienced not as a gift but as a threat. To be seen is to be rendered vulnerable. To be known is to risk annihilation.

This is particularly true in patients with schizoid or dissociative structures, where subjectivity has been organized around the fantasy of unreachability. Here, submission may emerge not as a desire to be controlled but as a wish to be held in asymmetry: to be near an other who will not demand reciprocity, who will not pierce the aestheticized membrane through which feeling becomes tolerable.

The paper proceeds through a clinical vignette, theoretical elaboration, and nuanced reflection. The cases are drawn from work with patients across gender and sexual orientation, but particular attention is paid to how erotic submission operates in the unconscious lives of gay men, whose developmental pathways often include early structures of erotic secrecy, stylization, and disavowal. Following thinkers such as Fairbairn (1952), Klein (1946), Loewald (1978a), and Stern (1997), and incorporating the ethical and phenomenological perspectives of Buber (1970), Levinas (1969), Derrida (1995), and Rank (1936), I offer a view of erotic submission not as a deviation from health, but as an adaptive and deeply ethical relational style.

We begin with a clinical moment that appears ordinary: a patient recounts a familiar erotic scenario. But the telling is dissociated, the atmosphere thick. Something is being shown, not just said. Something is being given over, without ever being asked for.

The Analyst's Position in the Scene

In treatments organized around erotic submission, the analyst is drawn into a field that resists coherence. We are offered something—attention, vulnerability, a performance of yielding—but that offering is often encrypted in disavowal. The patient may seem to be offering themselves, but not to us. Or not to us as we are, but as we are made to be within their structure: distant, neutral, powerful, or unreachable. This positioning can feel seductive or disorienting, but it is neither flirtation nor seduction in the ordinary sense. It is a dissociative maneuver, one that preserves asymmetry as a condition of safety.

One patient, Adrian, a gay man in his early thirties, exemplified this choreography. He came to treatment after a series of chaotic breakups. "I always end up the one who's too much," he told me in our first session. "Or not enough. Or both." His relationships were stormy, brief, and often organized around erotic intensity and emotional avoidance. What struck me early on was not his narrative but his presence. Adrian spoke in long, affectively flat monologues about sex. His descriptions were vivid, but detached—as though reporting on someone else's experience. "He bent me over the sink," he said once, glancing away. "It was hot, I think. I felt… used, but in a good way." He paused. "Or maybe not good. Just less alone."

It would have been easy to interpret this as compulsive repetition or to inquire into early trauma. But the room didn't feel compulsive—it felt curated. Adrian's tone, his gaze, the rhythmic pace of disclosure—it all felt choreographed. Not false, exactly. More like staged. A scene was being enacted, but I was unsure of my role. Was I the voyeur? The container? The uninvited witness?

These questions mattered less than the affective pull they evoked. I felt carefully positioned—drawn in, then held at a remove. When I leaned forward with gentle curiosity, he withdrew. When I responded neutrally, he escalated the detail. There was no right distance. I began to understand that my position in the room was part of the submission itself. He was giving himself over, but only on terms that guaranteed misrecognition.

Sullivan (1953) proposed that the analyst's "personality is the primary instrument of therapy." But in fields like this, the analyst's personhood is not simply brought in—it is captured and stylized. We are cast, not just transferred upon. The analyst becomes the object needed to sustain the patient's submission—an object whose very presence threatens to unmake the scene if it becomes too real.

This is where erotic submission diverges from masochism. In masochistic structures, the pain itself often holds meaning; in the dynamics I'm describing, it is the asymmetry and misalignment that sustains the psychic structure. To be touched, felt, and seen too clearly would disrupt the patient's aesthetic of offering. The analyst's challenge is to remain present without collapsing that structure. To not overidentify with the role assigned, nor disavow our implication.

In Adrian's case, I began to notice how carefully he watched my responses. He rarely looked at me directly, but he tracked my affect with precision. If I softened, he grew abstract. If I asked something too emotionally direct, he shifted into jokes. The room became a scene of stylized distance. Submission, here, was not about vulnerability—it was about control through misalignment.

Reich (1949) described character armor as the body's way of managing psychic danger. Adrian's submission functioned similarly—not as surrender, but as aesthetic protection. His bodily yielding was organized to keep psychic exposure at bay. If I entered too fully, the submission would collapse.

As treatment progressed, I began to sense when I was being invited closer—not through words, but through microshifts in atmosphere. One day, after a long silence, he said quietly, "Sometimes I think you know what I'm saying, even when I don't." I responded carefully, "That sounds both reassuring and unnerving." He didn't reply. But something in the room settled. The submission had not vanished. But it had become less stylized—less about misrecognition, more about proximity without collapse.

These moments offer a glimpse into the analyst's ethical position in such fields. We are not there to decode or disrupt. We are there to survive the choreography. To be the person who does not demand a more integrated offering. To be present inside the aesthetic—responsive but not invasive, human but not engulfing.

The analyst's presence, in this way, becomes a form of ethical containment. Not interpretation. Not empathy in the usual sense. But a kind of shared dissociation—reverent, restrained, willing to wait. Submission, in these treatments, is not a symptom to be resolved, but a structure to be accompanied. And that accompaniment begins with our willingness to be positioned—and to stay there.

Dissociation and the Affective Logic of Submission

Erotic submission is often narrated in cultural discourse as the dramatization of surrender, where one yields to the other's dominance. But in analytic work, submission rarely presents so cleanly. It is less about the positions taken in fantasy than about the emotional architecture that supports the scene. When patients present with dissociative submission, what we often witness is not a defense against agency—but the organization of psychic safety through affective deferral. Dissociation becomes a way of managing desire, not by erasing it, but by staging it at a distance.

Ava, a woman in her late forties, described her sexual life with clarity and poise. Twice divorced, she presented herself as independent, emotionally self-aware, and sexually open. Yet something in her narratives felt muted—distant not only in time, but in affect. She described past lovers with warmth, but also with a kind of aesthetic control. "I've always liked giving pleasure," she said. "It makes me feel… essential. But I don't always know what I feel during."

I asked gently, "During what, exactly?"

She paused. "During sex. I sort of float outside myself."

She smiled as she said it, but I could feel the room tighten. There was something mournful behind the ease. Ava's erotic life was rich with images and scenes, but affectively vacated. Pleasure had been organized around offering—not around reciprocity, not even around sensation. Submission was not something she sought—it was something that happened to her in stylized, unconscious choreography.

In this way, submission had become her form of dissociation.

Donnel Stern (1997) offers the concept of unformulated experience—affect and memory that are present in the psyche but not yet symbolized. In Ava's case, the erotic was not merely unformulated; it was aestheticized into unreachability. She described being present and absent at once: attending to the other's desire while holding her own in a frozen, peripheral register. Submission became a compromise—a way to sustain erotic contact without emotional rupture. The dissociation was not symptomatic; it was a structure of relating.

Unlike trauma-induced dissociation, which often entails a split from overwhelming affect, this form of erotic dissociation is ambient. It flows into the scene before contact begins. The patient may describe wanting intimacy while subtly organizing the space to prevent mutuality. The affective logic is not "I can't bear this," but "I can bear it only if I am not quite here."

With Ava, this choreography became clear in the third year of treatment, when she began dating someone new. "He's gentle," she said. "Too gentle," I asked what she meant. "He wants to know what I feel. In the moment. I freeze." I stayed silent. She added, "It's easier when I'm just his fantasy."

This was not masochism. It was survival through self-erasure. To become the fantasy was to disappear safely.

Here, submission is not about yielding control but about managing the unbearable tension of presence. To be in the erotic scene as oneself, with feeling, with need, would require too much exposure. The stylized choreography protects against that risk. It allows the erotic to unfold, but at a remove. The analyst's task is to hold that remove without collapsing it.

One afternoon, Ava described an encounter where she had pretended to climax. "It's easier," she said. "I didn't want to disappoint him." I asked softly, "And what about disappointing yourself?" She looked startled. Then, quietly, "I don't know what I want." We sat in silence. I could feel her discomfort, but also something else—relief.

That moment was not insight. It was an emergence. A flicker of unscripted presence inside a deeply habituated aesthetic.

These are the moments analytic work with submission makes possible—not interpretation, but contact. The analyst becomes the one who doesn't demand, doesn't seduce, doesn't withdraw. We become the ones who can tolerate the aesthetic without needing it to dissolve.

W. R. D. Fairbairn (1952) argued that internal object relations are shaped not by instinct but by the need for connection. When connection is dangerous, erotic life forms around what is survivable. In dissociative submission, the internal world organizes around asymmetry because mutuality feels annihilating.

But the longing for mutuality does not disappear. It remains, flickering at the edge of enactment. The patient may test the analyst through absence, control, or stylization—offering themselves just enough to be seen, but not enough to be felt. And when we fail to interpret that choreography as resistance, we may be drawn into subtle enactments of distance or intrusion.

Our work, then, is not to resolve the dissociation but to accompany its logic. To stay near the affect that cannot yet be felt, and to do so without turning away. Erotic submission, when understood through this lens, is not failure—it is form. A form that speaks when the patient cannot, that touches without contact, that offers survival in the language of giving-over.

The Analyst's Vulnerability in the Field

The erotic atmosphere in treatments shaped by dissociative submission does not remain at the level of the patient's material. It enters the analyst—sometimes subtly, sometimes with a disorienting pull. We find ourselves implicated in scenes we did not consent to, but cannot simply step out of. Our countertransference becomes saturated with contradiction: arousal and disinterest, protectiveness and withdrawal, irritation and grief. The analytic posture, in such treatments, is not one of mastery. It is one of vulnerability.

The analyst's task is not only to notice these dynamics, but to survive them—without retaliating, enacting, or disengaging. Erotic submission, when it unfolds in the transferential field, is often structured to pre-empt mutuality. The patient may position us as desired, feared, rejected, or erased—all in service of keeping the relational asymmetry intact. And yet, our very presence begins to destabilize that choreography. To remain embodied, receptive, and uncollapsed in the face of this stylization is to bear a kind of ethical tension—one that is somatic as much as it is interpretive.

With Adrian, the erotic field thickened as trust developed. But trust, in his case, meant the capacity to stage increasingly stylized scenes in which I was implicated as both witness and object. One day, after describing an emotionally numb hookup in granular detail, he looked at me and said, "You're not like that, are you?" I wasn't sure what "that" meant. I waited. He continued, "You seem like someone who doesn't need it to be anonymous." There was no question in his tone—only observation, and a touch of something else. Resentment? Admiration? Testing?

I said, "You're wondering about the kinds of intimacy I find tolerable."

He smiled, then shrugged. "Something like that."

I felt the room shift. Something personal had been offered—not about me, but about him. Yet I also felt the threat of collapse. If I answered directly, I risked stepping into his fantasy. If I ignored it, I risked repeating the erasure he already expected. My task was not to resolve the moment, but to remain in it.

Bollas (1992) reminds us that analysts are not blank screens; we are characters in the patient's world. But in dissociative erotic fields, the patient's internal world is orchestrated so intricately that it detaches from embodied experience. We are characters in a scene choreographed to protect the patient from what they simultaneously long for and dread: genuine presence. Our personhood becomes the site of tension—not because we are meant to disclose or perform, but because our aliveness threatens to pierce the aesthetic.

For queer analysts, this tension may be amplified. Our embodiment evokes recognition or fantasy that the patient cannot metabolize. As queer analysts in queer treatments, we are rarely neutral. We are too close to the patient's disavowed identification, too visible in our difference, too resonant in ways we cannot control. Even when unspoken, this proximity haunts the field.

In Adrian's case, my queerness became a kind of aperture through which the treatment unfolded. He never asked about it, but referenced it obliquely—mentioning "men like you," "your kind," or "guys who actually talk." Each phrase was a touch, an invocation, a test. My task was to remain tactile but bounded, responsive but intact.

This is not ordinary countertransference. It is a form of ethical receptivity that Donna Orange (2010) might describe as "empathic moral presence." We stay, not to interpret, but to make room—for feeling, for form, for flickers of relationality too fragile to be touched directly.

At times, I found myself retreating. I would notice my voice soften too much, or my silences stretch just slightly longer than needed. It wasn't just empathy—it was fear of rupturing something precious. Adrian's erotic field required a particular kind of containment: not blankness, but disciplined opacity. I had to remain human without becoming real. I had to be reachable without being touched.

These constraints are not failures. They are part of the terrain. The analyst's vulnerability in the field is not an obstacle to the work—it is the medium through which the work occurs. Our bodies, feelings, and uncertainties become sites of relational possibility. Not because we offer perfect attunement, but because we survive misrecognition without retaliation.

This is what makes the analyst's presence in these treatments so paradoxically powerful. We are not dominant, but we are felt as powerful—precisely because we are asked to remain visible while being refused. Erotic submission, in this sense, is a relational trial. Can the other remain without collapsing into demand? Can the analyst hold tension without trying to transform it?

When we do, something shifts—not in the patient's structure, but in the atmosphere. The choreography softens. The stylization loosens. The dissociation becomes less absolute.

And in that shift, mutuality—impossible, feared, disavowed—begins to flicker at the edge of the field.

Aestheticization and the Rhythm of Repair

What appears, at first, as repetition compulsion or relational resistance is often something more quietly sophisticated: the patient's aesthetic. Erotic submission, in dissociative structure, is not merely a re-enactment—it is a crafted form. A choreography of psychic preservation that allows feeling to be both near and held apart. These scenes are not accidents. They are poetic economies, designed to protect against annihilation by orchestrating the timing, tone, and proximity of contact.

In one session, Adrian recounted a hookup in which he asked the other man not to speak. "Words ruin it," he said. "When they talk, I start thinking about myself." He meant it literally. If the other became too real—too reciprocal—Adrian would become aware of himself not as scene-maker but as scene-subject. And that awareness was too much. His submission only worked if his subjectivity was oblique. His safety depended on a precisely managed rhythm of dissociation.

This is the aestheticization of psychic defense. But unlike theatricality, it is not aimed at the other's perception. It is aimed inward—toward the management of feeling. The erotic becomes a stylized rhythm: gesture, withholding, a curated cadence of approach and retreat. These rhythms are deeply private, often imperceptible to the patient themselves. But they form the scaffolding of what Stern (1997) calls "unformulated experience"—affective states that have never found relational traction.

Ava, too, lived inside this rhythm. Her submission took a more relationally responsive form: she attuned to the other so precisely that she disappeared into their need. "I'm a great lover," she once said. "If you don't care whether I'm there." It wasn't despairing—it was matter-of-fact. Her erotic aesthetic was built on minimizing her own presence. The rhythm was one of internal vanishings—precise and practiced.

Neither patient wished to be alone. But they had learned that being felt came at too great a cost. Erotic submission was a compromise: they could be present if their presence was partial. Aestheticization enabled them to be both seen and unseen, both desiring and insulated from the consequences of their desires.

What changes in treatment are not always structural? Often, it is the timing. The analyst does not interpret the aesthetic—we enter into its rhythm. We do not rupture the stylization—we breathe within it. Over time, the patient begins to tolerate small shifts: a pause where there was once a pivot, a silence that allows a feeling to arrive before it is deferred.

With Adrian, these shifts were imperceptible at first. He began to reference feelings indirectly—"I felt weird after," "It stayed with me"—phrases that had never surfaced before. They were not declarations of change. They were traces. Markers of a rhythm that had begun to slow, to open.

Reich (1949) suggested that the body holds what the psyche cannot. However, in these patients, the body has also undergone a transformation. The submission is not only psychic—it is somatic, choreographed in muscle and breath. The analyst's countertransference must track this, not as resistance, but as a signal. When the patient rushes through a moment or changes posture at a precise phrase—these are markers of the aesthetic. They tell us where feeling might live, if given time.

Repair does not come through confrontation. It comes through tempo. Through waiting with, bearing with, inhabiting the aesthetic without dissolving it. Over time, the stylization may soften—not as collapse, but as loosening. The patient may begin to improvise.

One day, Adrian ended a story mid-sentence. He shook his head. "I don't want to finish that one." I nodded. He looked at me. "You're not going to ask me to?" I said, "Not if stopping is what feels right."

He nodded again. We sat in silence. Something had changed. The scene had not resolved. But the rhythm had been his. That mattered.

Aestheticization is often pathologized in clinical literature—as if stylization is the enemy of truth. But for many patients, the aesthetic is their truth. It is the only form in which feeling can live. Our task is not to break it, but to learn its cadence. To become a co-witness to the rhythm through which affect emerges.

And when we do, something happens—not dramatic, not declarative. But human. The choreography becomes less about survival, more about contact. The submission remains, but it no longer conceals.

It begins to reveal.

Mutuality and the Aftermath of Stylization

For patients whose erotic structures are organized around dissociative submission, the prospect of mutuality is not merely unfamiliar—it is destabilizing. Their stylized modes of erotic being have evolved precisely to manage the unpredictability of contact. Mutuality is not the telos of their desire but the threat of its undoing. Yet, with time, treatment may bring them to its edge.

The work, then, must be careful. The analyst does not guide the patient "back" to mutuality, as if it were a developmental milestone to be recovered. Rather, we accompany the patient toward mutuality as a potential that emerges unevenly, haltingly, and with ambivalence.

In the fourth year of Adrian's treatment, he mentioned that he had begun dating someone more regularly. "It's not serious," he said. "We hang out, hook up, and keep it simple."

But a week later, he added, "He brought soup when I was sick. That was worse than any hookup."

I asked what made it worse. He said, "Because I didn't disappear."

The stylized distance that had governed his erotic life began to crack under the weight of ordinary care. The soup was not erotic. It was not performative. It was, in his terms, "too real." The man stayed the night, washed a few dishes, and left the next morning with a kiss on the forehead. Adrian felt exposed—not by what happened, but by what didn't. "There was nothing to hide behind," he said. "He was just… there."

Mutuality had brushed against him, and his response was not gratitude, but terror.

This is the aftermath of stylization. When the aesthetic softens, the feelings it was protecting come rushing forward. Not only fear, but shame, grief, even rage—at having lived so long without being met in this way. For the patient, the experience of care can feel violent. The analyst's role in these moments is not to reassure, but to remain.

Winnicott (1965) reminds us that the capacity to be alone develops only in the presence of another. But for patients like Adrian, being with another becomes possible only through stylized absence. To relinquish that aesthetic is to lose the form that has made relation survivable. The analyst must bear this grief without interpreting it away.

Ava experienced a similar rupture. After several years of treatment, she entered into a relationship that lasted more than a few months. "He sees me," she said once, then added, "but I don't know who he sees." Her submission no longer functioned. She felt herself both newly alive and utterly unmoored. "I don't know how to be with someone without becoming what they want."

That, too, was a form of emergence.

The analyst's task is to hold the aftermath of stylization—to bear the patient's confusion, grief, and newness without trying to resolve it too quickly. Mutuality must be allowed to feel as terrifying as dissociation once felt safe. It must be metabolized slowly, in fragments.

In the weeks after the soup, Adrian spoke less. But he stayed connected. He showed up. His narratives were thinner, but more proximate. "I don't know what I want," he said once, "but I don't want to ghost him." There was ambivalence, not defense. Longing, not choreography.

I said, "It seems like a part of you is staying, even if you're not sure how."

He looked up, uncertain. "Maybe. I didn't vanish this time."

Conclusion—The Discipline of Staying Near

In erotic fields shaped by dissociative submission, the analyst is not a distant observer of psychic life but an implicated participant in a highly curated relational aesthetic. What appears as absence or resistance often reveals itself to be a form—a carefully maintained choreography through which the patient makes contact without collapse. Submission, in this terrain, is not simply a defense. It is a grammar of proximity.

To work clinically in this space is to adopt a posture of disciplined accompaniment. The analyst does not demand clarification, does not rush integration, and does not assume that mutuality is the patient's destination. We learn to stay close to stylized distance, to hear the rhythm of withheld affect, and to tolerate misrecognition without needing to reclaim the transference. This is a position not of detachment but of ethical endurance.

What changes in treatment are rarely dramatic. It arrives in tempo: a softening, a slowing, a patient's glance that lingers half a second longer than before. These are not signs of resolution. They are signs of life returning to the scene. The stylization begins to loosen not because it is interpreted, but because it is held without intrusion.

In these moments, the analyst becomes less an agent of change and more a bearer of time. We offer continuity in a structure organized around aesthetic rupture. We become a witness who does not demand more than the patient can yet give—and in that restraint, something begins to breathe.

The patient may not name this change. It may never reach the language of insight. But it becomes visible in the atmosphere: in moments of stillness, in feelings that arrive without retreat, in the flickering emergence of want without strategy.

In this way, erotic submission does not dissolve—it deepens. It becomes something the patient can inhabit with slightly less fear. And the analyst, having stayed, becomes not the one who fixed it, but the one who made its unfolding survivable.

Epilogue: On Not Completing the Scene

Some treatments never resolve in the way we imagine they might. There is no moment of sudden coherence, no seamless integration of past and present, no clean shift from submission to sovereignty. Instead, what evolves is the patient's capacity to inhabit contradiction without fleeing it. To tolerate nearness without orchestrating every beat of the encounter.

What marks the work, in the end, is not what is said—but what is no longer required. The rehearsals grow less elaborate. The aesthetic control loosens. The analyst becomes less an object to be managed, more a presence to be tolerated.

This, too, is a form of change.

In the treatment of erotic submission, success does not lie in the undoing of stylization, but in its softening. Not in replacing performance with authenticity, but in allowing performance to be something other than a shield.

We do not complete the scene. We leave it slightly ajar.

And in that incompleteness, something freer begins to move.

Mutuality in these treatments is not a goal. It is a residue. A trace that begins to persist once the stylization becomes less necessary. The analyst does not push toward it—we wait, we witness, we stay. And when mutuality does arrive, it is not symmetrical. It is lived unevenly, with fear and longing braided together.

But it is real.

Part 2

Recursive Selves and Symbolic Reversal

4 The Original Paradox

This chapter explores paradox as a foundational structure of psychic life, rather than a disruption to be resolved. Drawing on myth, metapsychology, and contemporary psychoanalytic theory, it traces the recursive logic of contradiction from early creation myths through Freud, Klein, and Fairbairn, to the symbolic insights of Gödel and Derrida, and the clinical wisdom of Bion, Bollas, Ogden, and Levinas. At each turn, paradox is framed not as an error in cognition but as an expression of psychic truth—what cannot be fully symbolized yet must be lived. A clinical vignette brings these ideas to life in the analytic field, showing how paradox may be suffered, held, and gradually metabolized through a relationship. This chapter argues for an ethics of analytic presence that privileges accompaniment over resolution and proposes that psychoanalytic work is not a movement beyond paradox, but a deepening into its texture.

Introduction: The Paradox at the Beginning

Paradox is not merely a disruption in thought. It is a structure—an essential architecture of psychic life. From the earliest moments of being, the human subject encounters contradiction not as an anomaly, but as an atmosphere. To want and to fear, to reach and recoil, to speak and remain hidden—these are not pathologies. They are the conditions of our existence.

Psychoanalysis was born inside such contradictions. Freud's first patients spoke of memories that could not be remembered, truths that returned as symptoms, and desires they disavowed even as they enacted them. From the beginning, the unconscious was a paradoxical space: both known and unknown, hidden yet manifest, split and saturated.

And yet, psychoanalytic theory has often strained to resolve what cannot be resolved. Classical metapsychology tended toward structural explanations. Ego psychology aimed at adaptation and mastery. Even relational theories, for all their attention to multiplicity, have sometimes glossed over the impossibility at the heart of being with another: that to truly know the other is to risk losing them, and to preserve their alterity is to never fully understand.

This chapter does not aim to resolve paradox. It aims to dwell in it.

DOI: 10.4324/9781003715283-7

It argues that paradox is not an obstacle to be overcome, but a terrain to be navigated—symbolically, ethically, and clinically. It lives in the space between theory and practice, language and silence, containment and rupture. It appears in the split narratives of trauma, in the recursive loops of transference, in the oscillating demands placed on the analyst to be both subject and object, mirror and mystery.

To explore a paradox is also to question our own analytic reflexes. The urge to interpret, to integrate, to find coherence—these are important, but they can become premature closures. The most transformative moments in analytic work may not be those of insight, but of shared confusion: the moments when something resists articulation, and we agree to sit with it anyway.

This chapter unfolds through a series of recursive movements—theoretical, clinical, philosophical, and mythic. It begins with creation myths that cleave the world into being. It moves through Freud's split psyche, Klein's positions, and Fairbairn's internal objects. It turns through Gödel's mathematical limits and Derrida's slippages in signification. It listens with Bion, Bollas, and Ogden for what has not yet been symbolized. It pauses with Levinas at the ethical edge of witnessing. And it returns—as myth and psychic life always do—not to closure, but to deepened rhythm.

To write about paradox is to risk incoherence and to trust that something essential may be communicated even in the folds. This chapter does not offer a system. It offers a holding space—for readers, for patients, for ourselves.

Paradox does not need to be solved. It needs to be lived.

Creation Myths and the Cleaving of Origin

Every beginning requires a rupture. In mythological narratives across cultures, creation is not a gentle emergence—it is division. The world is born when the sky is split from the earth, when chaos is severed into form, when the primordial is cleaved into distinction. Creation begins not in wholeness, but in paradox: something must be destroyed for something else to appear.

In the Babylonian *Enuma Elish*, the god Marduk slays the primordial goddess Tiamat, and from her body, he fashions the heavens and earth. In Norse mythology, the world is built from the slain body of the giant Ymir. In the Hebrew *Genesis*, the spirit of God hovers over the deep and divides light from darkness, waters above from waters below. These are not stories of synthesis. They are dramas of severance.

Psychoanalytic theory has its own myths of origin—clinical rather than cosmological, but no less foundational. Freud's seduction theory, his later theory of repression, and his dual-drive model all hinge on the idea that the psyche emerges through conflict and division. The ego is not born whole; it is carved from the id by reality and prohibition. Identity itself is structured around internal splits.

This is why the earliest psychic life cannot be understood in terms of harmony. Melanie Klein, for instance, depicts the infant's first object relations not as unified attachments but as part–object relations split between the good and bad breast. In the *paranoid-schizoid position,* love and hate cannot be integrated; they are psychically torn apart to preserve coherence. It is only with development—and with mourning—that the *depressive position* becomes possible: a state in which contradictory feelings can be held within the same psychic space.

Creation, in this light, is not the emergence of unity, but the beginning of complexity. It is the origin of paradox—of simultaneous desire and dread, of longing and loss, of presence haunted by absence.

These myths offer more than metaphor. They speak to the internal architecture of psychic life. The subject does not begin as one. The subject begins as many—and must become one, only to split again.

This recursive tension lives at the heart of psychoanalytic work. Patients arrive with stories of rupture—traumatic, developmental, relational. These ruptures are not merely past events. They are living realities. The self remains split. The analytic task is not to stitch it closed, but to create a space where contradiction can be borne.

To work with paradox, then, is to engage in a kind of re-creation. Analysis is not about returning to a mythical wholeness. It is about forming something new from the fragments—not through synthesis, but through symbolic bearing. The psyche is not unified; it is assembled. And that assembly requires room for what cannot be resolved.

In myth, the world is made from a corpse. In analysis, the self is made from its own psychic remains—from what was split, denied, and broken. This is not bleak. It is sacred. The cleaving is not the end of coherence. It is its beginning.

Freud's Divided Mind and the Birth of the Unconscious

Freud never unified the mind. He split it.

In his early studies of hysteria, he observed that certain memories and affects were not merely forgotten—they were cordoned off, inaccessible to consciousness but still active. These repressed elements did not vanish. They returned in disguise: in symptoms, dreams, slips, and enactments. Thus, the unconscious was born not as a poetic idea, but as a necessity—a domain of experience that could not be integrated yet continued to shape thought and behavior.

Freud's topographical model cast the mind into conscious, preconscious, and unconscious territories. Later, his structural model introduced the id, ego, and superego—psychic agencies defined less by location than by function and conflict. In both schemas, what remains constant is division. The psyche, for Freud, is not a harmony of parts. It is a battleground.

Repression was the first mechanism he named, but the logic of contradiction was already embedded. The symptom is itself a paradox: a compromise formation that expresses both wish and defense. The dream is another: a fulfillment of desire that conceals its fulfillment. The very language of the unconscious is ambivalent—driven by condensation, displacement, and negation. It says what it means by not saying it.

Freud's case histories are filled with such paradoxes. The woman who coughs to silence her desire. The man who blinds himself to see. The patient who forgets in order to remember. These are not poetic turns; they are the core mechanics of psychic life.

In *Beyond the Pleasure Principle*, Freud ventured further into paradox, proposing that alongside the drive for pleasure and cohesion lay a death drive—a compulsion toward repetition, stasis, and return. This was not a regression in theory but a deepening. Freud was beginning to glimpse that contradiction is not a failure of the mind. It is its structure.

What Freud could not yet fully theorize was the intersubjective field in which these paradoxes unfold. He saw the patient's suffering, but he often cast himself as the decipherer, the one who knew. Later analysts would reframe the analytic situation as a co-constructed field, where the analyst's subjectivity is implicated, where countertransference is not noise but data, and where the encounter itself becomes the medium through which paradox is lived.

But Freud laid the groundwork. He insisted that truth and conflict are not opposites. That we can want what we fear, know what we deny, love what we hate. He taught us to listen not for coherence, but for contradiction—to follow the symptom back to its double meanings.

If Klein and Fairbairn would later map these paradoxes developmentally, and Bion and Bollas would attend to their unformulated residues, it was Freud who first gave them a language. A language already split.

To read Freud today is not to find a unified theory. It is to find a mind wrestling with its own contradictions—returning to the same questions with new formulations, circling what cannot be resolved. His theories evolve, break down, and reconfigure. This recursive movement mirrors the psyche itself: always returning, always divided, always in search of a form that can hold what does not yet make sense.

Klein and Fairbairn: The Developmental Life of Splitting

If Freud introduced the concept of the paradoxical unconscious, Klein and Fairbairn provided it with a developmental history. They moved psychoanalysis inward—into the early life of the infant, where the psyche is forged not only in drives, but in relationships. For both theorists, the self is not a given. It is shaped by love, by loss, by failure, and by repair. And its early life is split.

Melanie Klein's depiction of infancy is steeped in contradiction. In the earliest months, she proposed, the infant is not in relationship with whole objects but with part-objects—not with "mother" but with "the breast." These objects are imbued with intense affective valence. The good breast soothes; the bad breast frustrates. When the infant cannot integrate these experiences, they are split: one idealized, the other persecutory.

This is the *paranoid-schizoid position*—a term that confounds because it is not pathological in itself. It is a developmental state, marked by primitive defenses like splitting, projection, and idealization. The world is experienced in absolutes. There is no both/and. Only good or bad, safe or threatening. The psyche preserves coherence by fragmenting it.

Only later—with maturation and containment—does the infant enter the *depressive position*. Here, ambivalence becomes thinkable. The good and bad breasts are recognized as aspects of the same mother. Love and hate can coexist. Guilt and mourning emerge. The self, no longer split, becomes capable of concern.

Paradoxically, this integration is a loss. The certainty of absolutes gives way to the ambiguity of reality. And it is this loss—this confrontation with contradiction—that makes psychic life possible.

Fairbairn, working independently, offered a related but distinct account. He rejected Freud's pleasure principle as the core motivator of psychic life, insisting instead that the self is driven to relate. Libido is object-seeking, not pleasure-seeking. The child does not desire satisfaction; they desire connection.

But when connection is traumatic—when the parent is inconsistent, intrusive, or abandoning—the child faces an impossible dilemma. They need the object, but the object hurts. In response, the psyche splits. The "good" aspects of the parent are internalized in one part–object relationship; the "bad" in another. The self, too, fragments. One part relates to the idealized object. Another bonds with the rejecting one. A third retreats into isolation.

These internal object relations form the basis of later psychic structure. They are not memories. They are ongoing relationships within the self. And they are saturated with paradox: the child who hates the parent they still long to please; the internal object that soothes and shames in the same breath.

Both Klein and Fairbairn show that splitting is not a failure. It is an achievement—a way of organizing experience that would otherwise overwhelm. The problem arises not in the existence of splitting, but in its rigidity. When contradictory affects cannot be integrated, the self remains fractured. The analytic task is to create a space where these divisions can soften, where the persecutory and idealized can be felt in proximity.

But this softening is not an interpretive feat. It is a relational one. The analyst becomes a new object—one who does not retaliate or abandon, who can be hated and still remain, who can survive idealization without collapse. Over time, this relational field allows for the symbolic possibility of holding contradiction.

Klein and Fairbairn help us see that paradox is not simply a matter of abstract thought. It is inscribed in the very development of the self. The infant does not move from unity to multiplicity. They begin in fragmentation and must work—with another—to bear it.

Gödel and Derrida: Incompleteness and Slippage

Paradox is not confined to the clinic or the developmental field. It is embedded in the structure of logic and meaning itself. With Kurt Gödel and Jacques Derrida, we enter the symbolic domain—where contradiction is not the exception but the rule, and where every act of signification carries the trace of what it cannot contain.

Gödel's incompleteness theorems shook the foundation of mathematical certainty. In essence, he demonstrated that any sufficiently complex formal system will contain propositions that are true but cannot be proven within that system. There will always be statements that exceed the logical scaffolding meant to hold them. The system, in attempting to define all truth, becomes structurally open—and structurally incomplete.

This is not merely a mathematical insight. It is a philosophical one. It tells us that coherence is never total, that closure generates its own gaps. Every structure carries a remainder—something unprovable, unsymbolizable, outside. Paradox, in Gödel's model, is not a breakdown. It is intrinsic.

Derrida, working in a different register, came to a similar conclusion about language. In his concept of *différance*—a neologism combining difference and deferral—Derrida shows that meaning is never fully present. Every sign refers to another sign. Every word points beyond itself. The signified is always postponed. There is no final arrival, no foundational ground. Language is a system of gaps, slippages, and ghostly traces.

Where Gödel reveals a limit internal to logical systems, Derrida reveals a dispersal internal to signification. What they share is a commitment to the paradoxical structure of meaning: every effort to fix truth re-introduces instability. Every attempt to say the thing misses it—and this very missing is what allows language to function at all.

For the analyst, these insights are not academic. They are clinical. We encounter them each time a patient reaches for language and recoils. Each time, an interpretation feels both right and evasive. The patient who says, "I don't know what I'm feeling, but I know it matters" is voicing something that cannot yet be symbolized—something that hovers at the edge of expression, where the trace exceeds the sign.

This is where interpretation, though necessary, can become premature. When the analyst rushes to name what is still forming, they risk collapsing the symbolic space that holds the paradox. The patient may nod in agreement while withdrawing internally. Or they may protest without knowing why. The interpretation, like Gödel's unprovable proposition, is true but unworkable—not because it's wrong, but because the structure is not yet ready to receive it.

Clinically, this often manifests as a kind of semantic drift. The patient circles a theme—abandonment, shame, annihilation—but every articulation feels slightly askew. The analyst senses something vital underneath, but it slips each time it is spoken. The work, then, is not to arrive at a coherent narrative, but to stay with the slippage. To honor the symptom as a site of paradox, where the unspeakable is half-spoken, and the half-spoken is saturated with more than it can contain.

This view resonates with Freud's idea of condensation and displacement in dreams—processes that encode contradiction in form. But Derrida takes this further: the very condition for meaning is the failure of full presence. Interpretation becomes not the revelation of a hidden core, but a dance with the remainder.

And so, paradox again becomes a structure, not a disruption. The analyst is not a decoder, but a listener to the gaps—a reader of what is missing. The symptom, the silence, the misstatement: each is a portal to something that will not appear in full.

This is not a reason to give up on interpretation. It is a call to refine our listening. To track not only what is said, but the moment when meaning unravels. To hear, in the analytic field, the echo of Gödel's unprovable truths and Derrida's endless deferrals.

In doing so, we shift from the fantasy of insight-as-resolution to the ethics of staying-with. Paradox cannot be interpreted away. But it can be lived through. And in that living, something symbolic begins to form—not as a final word, but as a holding pattern for what exceeds containment.

In the next section, we return more directly to the clinical field through the work of Bion, Bollas, and Ogden—theorists who help us sit with what has not yet been dreamed, thought, or named, and who remind us that paradox lives not only in theory, but in the texture of presence.

Bion, Bollas, and Ogden: The Symbolic Life of the Not-Yet-Known

If Klein and Fairbairn show us how the self develops through fragmentation and splitting, Bion, Bollas, and Ogden take us deeper into the experiential texture of unformed psychic life. Their work gives us a language for what has not yet taken symbolic shape—for states that precede meaning but insist on being felt.

Wilfred Bion described the infant as bombarded by unprocessed sense impressions, raw affects, and proto-experiences. These "beta elements" are undigested fragments that the infant cannot yet think. The caregiver's task—and later, the analyst's—is to perform the *alpha function*: to receive these fragments, metabolize them, and return them in a form that can be symbolized. This is not just a relational act; it is a symbolic one. The origins of thought, for Bion, lie in the transformation of the inchoate into the thinkable.

When containment fails, the consequences are profound. The infant is left with nameless dread—an experience of catastrophic fragmentation that cannot be assimilated. In analysis, we encounter this not only in psychotic states, but in the quiet presence of what cannot yet be said. The patient may arrive and speak fluently, but the analyst feels something weighty in the room—an emotional residue that exceeds language. These are the traces of beta elements still circulating, waiting to be thought.

Bollas builds on this with his concept of the *unthought known*—those early relational experiences that were never symbolized but nonetheless shape the internal world. These are not repressed because they were never fully formed. They live in gesture, affective tone, relational style—in how the patient leans away at the moment of contact or repeats a pattern they cannot name.

The *unthought known* cannot be interpreted into existence. It must be midwifed into form. This often requires a kind of interpretive restraint—a willingness on the analyst's part to feel with rather than speak for. The analyst becomes a container not of insight, but of atmospheric pressure: a presence capable of allowing the unformulated to emerge without suffocating it in language.

Ogden extends this tradition with his concept of the *undreamt dream*—experiences that have not yet been dreamed because they are not yet thinkable. These are the psychic materials that lie beyond even repression. They have not been forgotten; they have not yet happened in psychic life. The analytic space, then, becomes a place where dreaming can begin: not in the sense of wish fulfillment, but in the sense of psychic integration. Dreaming becomes a metaphor for symbolizing what had remained unlivable.

In the consulting room, we encounter the undreamt in silence, in confusion, in affect that has no narrative. A patient may say, "I feel like something is wrong, but I don't know what." Or they may say nothing at all, and the analyst feels a tightness in their own chest, a heaviness that cannot be named. These moments are not gaps in communication. They are the field in which the psyche begins to gather itself.

The analyst's task is not to decode but to dream alongside. This is not passive. It is a deeply participatory stance: to offer a mind capable of holding contradiction without foreclosure, capable of sustaining ambiguity without collapse. It is to act as a second skin for the psyche until its own symbolic capacities can emerge.

All three theorists offer us ways to think about paradox not as an interpretive dilemma, but as a structural necessity. What cannot be symbolized remains active. What cannot be thought returns in the body, in the atmosphere, in the relational field.

The presence of the analyst becomes the transitional space through which the unthought can become thinkable. This is not a linear process. It is recursive, nonverbal, and often painful. But it is also the space of possibility—the space where paradox can be lived, felt, and eventually dreamed.

In the next section, we move from the symbolic to the ethical—from the analyst as transformer of meaning to the analyst as witness to what exceeds symbolization altogether. With Levinas, we enter the paradox of responsibility: how to respond to what cannot be contained.

Levinas and the Paradox of Witnessing

In the work of Emmanuel Levinas, we encounter a radical rethinking of subjectivity—one that does not begin in autonomy, but in relation. For

Levinas, the self is not sovereign. It is summoned. The face of the other interrupts the self's mastery and calls it into responsibility. And yet, this ethical relation is not symmetrical. The self is commanded to respond to the other—not because it understands, but because it cannot.

This is the paradox at the heart of witnessing: one is asked to respond to a suffering one cannot fully know. To be present to an alterity that escapes symbolization. To bear an ethical responsibility without the guarantee of comprehension. For Levinas, this asymmetry is not a flaw—it is the condition of ethics itself.

Psychoanalysis, particularly in its relational and intersubjective forms, has increasingly recognized the centrality of witnessing. But this witnessing is often misunderstood as recognition, as seeing and being seen. Levinas offers something more unsettling: to witness is not to master, but to be undone. The other's suffering disrupts the self's coherence. The analyst is not a mirror, but a site of ethical disturbance.

In the analytic encounter, this takes many forms. A patient recounts a trauma that cannot be fully symbolized. They speak haltingly or not at all. The room is filled with absence, with what cannot be said. The analyst feels pulled—to name it, to soothe it, to understand. But none of these responses is adequate. What is required is a different kind of presence: one that does not consume the patient's experience with interpretation, but holds it in its opacity.

Levinas insists that the self must make space for what cannot be assimilated. This is profoundly difficult in analysis, where the tools of meaning-making are so central. But sometimes, interpretation is too much. The patient does not need to be understood. They need to be accompanied.

This reframes our understanding of containment. It is not merely a function—it is an ethical act. To contain is to suffer with, to remain open to what the patient cannot yet symbolize. It is to stand in proximity to the unbearable without retreating into knowledge or technique.

Analytic training often emphasizes attunement, empathy, and reflection. But Levinas reminds us that true ethical witnessing may exceed all of these. It is not empathy that constitutes the ethical relation, but exposure. The analyst, like the Levinasian subject, is exposed to the patient's suffering—not to master it, but to refuse its erasure.

In practice, this might mean sitting in silence, even when words feel demanded. It might mean tolerating the analyst's own helplessness, frustration, or despair. It may mean accepting that the analytic space is not a site of repair, but rather a site of accompaniment.

This does not mean giving up on symbolization. But it means letting it emerge from the field, rather than imposing it. The paradox of witnessing is that the more we try to grasp, the more we risk losing the very thing we are trying to hold. To witness, then, is to hold without grasping. To stay near without consuming.

Levinas's ethics refuses resolution. It insists that the self is always in excess of itself, always summoned by a demand it cannot fulfill. This is deeply consonant with the analytic process, where the analyst is called to listen to what they cannot fix, to accompany what cannot be mended, to lend structure without closure.

In the next section, we will shift from theory to structure—examining how different levels of personality organization shape a patient's capacity to tolerate paradox. With McWilliams and Kernberg, we will explore how psychic structure mediates the experience of contradiction—and how the analyst must titrate paradox according to what the patient can bear.

Structural Tolerance for Paradox

If paradox is the atmosphere of psychic life, not all structures breathe it equally. The capacity to tolerate contradiction—to hold ambivalence, to live with split feelings, to endure ambiguity—is not simply a function of maturity or insight. It is shaped by the deeper architecture of the psyche: the level of personality organization that determines what kinds of experiences can be symbolized, held, and metabolized.

Otto Kernberg and Nancy McWilliams offer frameworks for understanding these structures. Drawing from object relations theory, Kernberg identifies three broad levels of personality organization: neurotic, borderline, and psychotic. Each is marked by differing degrees of identity integration, defensive style, and reality testing. McWilliams, in parallel, describes these levels with a clinical texture that attends to the lived experience of affect regulation, relational capacity, and symbolic function.

At the neurotic level, the self is relatively cohesive. Defenses are predominantly repression-based. The patient may struggle with conflict, guilt, and ambivalence, but they can reflect on these difficulties. Paradox is uncomfortable, even painful, but it is not shattering. The analytic work at this level often involves making implicit conflict explicit—interpreting the contradiction so that it can be symbolized and integrated.

At the borderline level, the psychic terrain is more volatile. Splitting is a dominant defense. The self and others are experienced in polarized terms: all-good or all-bad, idealized or devalued. Ambiguity is dangerous because it threatens psychic cohesion. The same object cannot be both loving and frustrating—to accept this would feel like annihilation. Here, paradox is not just distressing; it is intolerable. The analyst becomes either savior or persecutor, and the patient moves between these poles with little sense of continuity.

In these cases, interpretation may be premature. The analyst's task is not to resolve the contradiction but to survive it. To remain present through the oscillations. To become an object that can eventually be held in paradox—not perfect, not hated, but real. This requires immense emotional discipline: to resist the urge to defend, retaliate, or withdraw. The analyst must titrate paradox to the level the patient can bear.

At the psychotic level, symbolic function itself may be compromised. Words lose their anchoring capacity. Reality testing is fragile or absent. Paradox here becomes something else entirely—not a structure to be endured, but a collapse into confusion. The work at this level is slow, often nonverbal. The analyst's presence may serve as a kind of scaffolding for psychic organization. Interpretation, when it comes, is more about rhythm and repetition than insight. The paradox cannot be named, but it can be shared.

Even within more integrated structures, pockets of fragmentation persist. A patient may function neurotically in most areas and regress to borderline or psychotic organization under relational stress. These shifts are especially common when early trauma has been disavowed or unmentalized. The analyst must learn to listen not only to the words but to the structure from which they emerge. What feels like a contradiction to the analyst may feel like annihilation to the patient.

This structural perspective helps us understand why some patients find paradox enlivening while others experience it as unbearable. The analyst's sensitivity to these thresholds is a clinical art—one that cannot be dictated by theory alone. It requires attunement to tone, tempo, and the implicit emotional logic of the session.

Importantly, structural capacity is not fixed. It can be expanded—slowly, relationally, over time. The analytic relationship becomes a crucible for tolerating more. The analyst models a mind that can hold contradiction without rupture, that can be both firm and permeable, reflective, and affectively alive. This is not containment as passivity, but as ethical vitality.

What we call growth, in psychoanalysis, may often be nothing more—and nothing less—than the increased capacity to live inside paradox without resorting to defense or collapse. To let the self stretch across contradiction and remain intact.

In the next section, we shift from theory back into the clinical encounter. Through a detailed case vignette, we will witness paradox not as an idea, but as a structure lived in real time—something enacted, suffered, and gradually made symbolically bearable.

Clinical Vignette: A Paradox Lived in the Field

Jacob came into treatment shortly after a series of relational ruptures. He was in his early forties, highly articulate, and self-identified as psychologically sophisticated. His intake forms were dense with language about boundaries, trauma, and emotional labor. He described his previous therapists as "well-meaning but naive" and made it clear he was looking for something deeper. "I don't want symptom relief," he told me. "I want someone who can sit with what's real."

Despite this, our work began with an almost antiseptic quality. Jacob intellectualized with great fluency. He narrated his past with an uncanny detachment, describing childhood neglect, the emotional absence of his mother, and the cruelty of a father who oscillated between indulgence and humiliation. But he told these stories with a kind of tonal flatness—like quoting a textbook on himself.

And then, as sometimes happens, the rupture came suddenly.

It was a session like any other. He was recounting an interaction with a friend who had "misread" his silence as disinterest. He looked at me and said, "You're doing that right now, aren't you?" There was a shift in the room—subtle, but immediate. His posture changed. His voice dropped. "You think you understand me," he said, "but you're just like the rest. You want me to be vulnerable, and then you recoil when it actually happens."

In that moment, I felt two things simultaneously: the impulse to clarify (I hadn't recoiled) and the pull to retreat (it felt like I had). His words landed like a projection, but also like a truth.

This was not a misunderstanding. It was an enactment—one shaped by paradox. He both longed to be seen and was certain he could not be. He demanded closeness and then attacked it the moment it appeared. To engage was to risk intrusion. To withdraw was to confirm abandonment. There was no position that did not replicate the trauma.

My task was not to resolve this, but to stay with it. I said, quietly, "It feels like being close is both something you want — and something that feels dangerous when it happens."

He looked at me, stunned. "That's the first real thing you've said," he whispered. And then: "Don't ruin it."

I said nothing. The silence that followed was full—heavy, but not deadened. It was a silence that held contradiction, a silence that did not foreclose.

Over the next few weeks, these moments repeated. Sometimes he would arrive and speak with great intimacy, only to disappear for a month. Other times, he would rage about how little I understood, and then fall silent in the same breath. Each time, the paradox returned: he wanted me to witness his pain, but not name it. He needed me to stay, but did not expect trust. He feared engulfment and abandonment equally.

This was not resistance. It was structured. The very idea of a reliable other was overdetermined—saturated with memory and threat. The analytic task was not to dismantle the paradox, but to survive it alongside him. To be reshaped by it.

As the work deepened, Jacob began to narrate fewer "insights" and more feelings. He said things like, "I know you're here, but I keep waiting for you to vanish." Or "I hate how much this matters." These were not linear progressions. They were recursive movements—circling the same wounds with new symbolic capacity.

One day, he arrived and sat quietly for nearly the entire session. At the end, he said, "I didn't want to talk. I just needed you to see that I showed up anyway."

It was a small moment. But it shimmered with meaning. The paradox had not been solved, but held unresolved. And in that holding, something shifted: not a resolution, but a new rhythm. A different way of breathing inside contradiction.

Jacob remains in treatment. Our work continues in fits and loops, in retreats and returns. The paradox is still present—but now it is livable. It no longer splits the field. It gives it shape.

The Return: Recursion, Myth, and the "Always Already There"

Paradox does not resolve. It returns.

This chapter began with myth—with the cleaving of origin and the division that gives rise to being. It winds back now not to conclude, but to re-affirm that the psyche does not unfold in straight lines. Psychic life circles. It re-encounters what was never integrated. It repeats not as failure, but as structure.

Freud's theory of repetition compulsion was the first analytic articulation of this return. The subject is drawn to re-stage what could not be symbolized, as if the doing-again might make it knowable. But the return is not always compulsion. Sometimes it is the very shape of symbolization. The psyche does not heal by moving away from contradiction, but by returning to it differently—newly metabolized, newly held.

This is the rhythm of recursive experience: the loop that does not circle back to the same place, but to the same place changed. In psychoanalysis, this is the structure of growth. A session may echo a prior rupture, but the analyst now holds it differently. The interpretation may not land at first, but later returns, inflected by time. The patient may leave and return, leave and return—each time closer to something bearable.

In this, psychoanalysis shares something with myth, poetry, and mysticism: a refusal of linear resolution. The recursive is not regressive. It is transformative. To return is not to relapse, but to remember with more of the self present.

The structure of the chapter mirrors this. From origin myths to symbolic function, from fragmentation to containment, from theory to case and back again—the movement is not additive, but spiral. This is not merely a literary choice. It is an epistemological one. Paradox cannot be captured in a single frame. It must be turned, re-encountered, re-heard.

And beneath this structure lies something more ancient: the sense that truth, when it finally arrives, was always there. In mystical traditions—particularly in Eastern thought—truth is not discovered but uncovered. The self does not gain it, but awakens to it. It is *always already there*. This phrase, drawn into Western philosophy by Derrida and others, captures the eerie familiarity of deep insight. The patient says, "I think I've always known this." And perhaps they have.

Michael Eigen describes this kind of knowing as *felt contact with being*—a moment where the psyche brushes up against something it never quite forgot. Mark Epstein, drawing from Buddhist psychology, writes of insight not as acquisition but as *recognition*—a return to the experiential field beneath defenses.

These moments shimmer. They cannot be forced. They emerge when the field is ready to hold them. And often, they are born in paradox: in the moment when the patient both trusts and distrusts, both clings and recoils, both yearns and resists. The analytic task is not to reconcile, but to stay long enough for the return to become tolerable.

The recursive structure of psychic life echoes in the structure of language itself. Just as Gödel showed that every formal system contains truths it cannot prove, and Derrida that every sign defers its own completion, so too does the psyche hold within it what it cannot fully symbolize—and what it nevertheless must return to again and again.

This is the return of the *undreamt dream*. The repetition of the *unthought known*. The reactivation of the unbearable truth that seeks a different witness. It is not a linear movement toward health, but a spiral around meaning, density, and presence.

Psychoanalysis, at its best, is a practice of staying-with—a ritual of return. The analyst does not move the patient forward, but accompanies them back: back into the mythic cleaving, the structural split, the symbolic field, the witnessing gaze. And each time, if the field can hold it, something new is born—not as a replacement, but as a re-iteration with a difference.

To work with paradox is to relinquish the fantasy of cure. It is to enter a rhythm of encounter, rupture, and return. And it is to believe that even in fragmentation, even in contradiction, something always remains—something waiting to be held.

5 The Madonna–Whore–Hologram

Erotic Dissociation, Affective Survival, and the Analyst's Double Position

This paper introduces the *Madonna–whore–hologram* as a clinical structure that reframes erotic dissociation not as pathology, but as an aesthetic of survival. Emerging in treatments marked by shame, secrecy, and disrupted witnessing—especially with queer male patients—the hologram describes an atmosphere in which erotic life becomes stylized across mutually incompatible identifications. The patient does not merely split objects; they refract time, presence, and affect. Drawing from object relations theory, dissociation literature, and post-structural ethical thought, the paper explores how the analyst is drawn into a shimmering field of erotic contradiction—cast as too pure to touch, too knowing to approach, too present to tolerate. In this clinical terrain, reverie becomes a matter of survival, and analytic presence becomes a devotional task. Through clinical vignettes and theoretical meditation, the paper considers how erotic opacity may be held without demand, how disavowal becomes a form of protection, and how the analyst's willingness to be misrecognized without retreat may offer the patient an experience of contact that does not collapse their structure. The hologram, when reverently inhabited, becomes not an obstacle to intimacy, but its fractured and flickering threshold.

Introduction

Many of us encounter patients whose erotic lives shimmer just out of reach. They describe sex without feeling it, narrate desire as performance, or speak from within relational scripts that seem uninhabited. In these treatments, something is present but displaced—held in the atmosphere more than in words. The analyst feels it first: not always as arousal, but as a shift in breath, a fog in the room, a pulse of unease. The erotic appears not as fantasy or confession, but as a field condition—a shimmering structure of partial disclosure and dissociative style.

This paper offers one name for that structure: the *Madonna–whore–hologram*. The term emerged not as a diagnosis but as a metaphor—a way to describe a particular dissociative aesthetic in which erotic vitality is split across affective positions that cannot coexist. Patients navigate mutually exclusive

DOI: 10.4324/9781003715283-8

identifications: the adored but untouchable, the degraded but desired, the spectator, and the absent self. Unlike Freud's (1912) formulation—where love and desire are neurotically separated—the hologram is not reducible to an intrapsychic split. It is a field phenomenon. A structure of presence and absence. A protection built through stylization.

This chapter may be understood, in part, as an extension of Christopher Bollas's (1992) reflections on "cruising in the homosexual arena," where the erotic charge arises not from mutual recognition, but from the object's resistance to full knowing. Drawing on psychoanalytic and literary motifs, Bollas illuminates how desire is often sustained through opacity—the other must remain just beyond comprehension in order to magnetize fantasy, projection, and transference. When the other becomes too legible, when their edges sharpen into clarity, the erotic spell may falter, and the object dissolves into the ordinary. The structure I trace here shares that dynamic tension: the Madonna–whore constellation similarly hinges on distance as erotic infrastructure. The Madonna, overexposed to moral proximity, may become de-eroticized; the whore, though sexually legible, often resides outside relational depth. In both modes, desire is preserved through a protective dialectic of withholding. As the subject approaches either intimacy or intelligibility, longing either gives way to defense or collapses altogether. It is this recursive balance—between psychic vividness and relational elusiveness—that gives the structure its holographic quality. The desired other appears fully formed in the mind's eye, yet remains physically ungraspable, allowing dissociated fragments to cohere against the surface of a curated, unreachable figure.

What I have come to understand, particularly in work with gay male patients, is that this structure is often developmental. The erotic self forms under conditions of secrecy—marked by projection, disavowal, and premature aestheticization. The hologram is not simply defensive; it is **devotional**. A dissociative architecture that holds unbearable contradiction until it becomes livable.

Drawing from Winnicott, Fairbairn, Eigen, Stern, and Levinas—as well as Derrida, Buber, Sedgwick, and Rank—I explore how the hologram functions as both a symptom and a gesture. Through clinical vignettes, I demonstrate how the analyst's body, reverie, and ethical restraint become integral to the therapeutic terrain. The paper unfolds as a meditation on how we bear erotic misrecognition without correction, how we hold the shimmer without collapsing it into clarity, and how our own queerness, if held with care, becomes part of what allows the patient to risk presence.

The Shimmering Field

Julian arrived with the confidence of someone who had been in therapy before. He was articulate, reflexive, and fluent in the language of insight. A gay man in his thirties, he described himself—dryly—as "good at therapy." His presenting concern was familiar: "I keep choosing men who won't choose me." But beneath that refrain, something else stirred—less nameable, more ambient. There was desire, clearly, but it floated in the room, dislocated from affect, stylized, oddly unreachable.

Julian recounted sexual encounters with precision, but little felt presence. He could narrate roles, gestures, and scripts—but not emotions. "Used, I guess? Or maybe that's what I wanted," he'd say, with a smile that pre-empted interpretation. He spoke of longing, but only in the past tense. He described sex without embodiment. The erotic had been flattened—not numbed entirely, but **aestheticized into distance**.

Over time, a structure revealed itself. Julian didn't just struggle with intimacy—he rotated through relational positions that canceled each other out. Men who were sexually available were too unsafe to feel with. Men who evoked yearning became untouchable. Tenderness threatened collapse. Sex was available, but he left his body. "I don't like being touched," he said. "But I like being wanted."

The analytic atmosphere mirrored this pattern. I found myself pulled into contradictory identifications: the one to impress, the one to seduce, the one too sacred to spoil. Some days I felt cast as the idealized mother; other days, the indifferent trick. Occasionally, I felt degraded, then erased. These were not transference fragments to be interpreted—they were roles into which I was projected and held. The erotic field shimmered: charged, flickering, unstable. Alive—but unreachable.

This is where the *hologram* metaphor emerged—not to diagnose, but to **articulate a clinical aesthetic.** Unlike a simple split, a hologram generates an image that appears whole from certain angles—but vanishes when approached too directly. Julian's erotic field operated similarly. Its coherence was conditional, its affective truth encrypted in stylization. Move toward it too directly, and it dissolved. Stay outside it, and it flickered in repetition.

What we were in the presence of was not simply defense—it was structure. The erotic had been shaped through a history of unmirrored desire. To feel, for Julian, was not just risky—it was unthinkable. He needed the aesthetic distance of enactment to tolerate proximity at all.

Winnicott's (1965) line kept returning to me: "It is a joy to be hidden, but a disaster not to be found." Julian's erotic life had been built on the necessity of hiding. But the disaster of being found too soon—or too clearly—had already been lived. What the hologram offered was something else entirely: not contact, not absence, but a protected shimmer of something that might someday become contact.

As his analyst, I learned to stay near the flicker without grasping it. I did not interpret the split. I did not try to integrate desire and shame. I bore the tension of erotic incoherence. Over time, Julian began to speak differently—not clearly, but haltingly. "I think I want someone to know me," he said once, "but I'm terrified it'll kill the wanting."

That line became a threshold. Not because it was revelatory, but because it marked a shift: from performance to presence, from ritualization to uncertainty. He hadn't stepped through the hologram. But he'd gestured to it—and allowed me to remain near.

Erotic Reverie and the Analyst's Affective Body

When erotic experience is dissociated, it rarely arrives through speech. It arrives through tone, posture, repetition—through the analyst's body. In treatments like Julian's, where desire cannot yet be directly felt or voiced, the analytic space becomes a site of atmospheric saturation. The patient speaks, but something else accumulates. The erotic becomes environmental—*sensed rather than said*.

Michael Eigen (1986) describes reverie not as a tool, but as a state—an openness to being altered by the unspeakable. In Julian's sessions, reverie wasn't a technique. It was survival. I often left feeling dazed, touched by something unspoken, or oddly ashamed—not because of what had been said, but because of what had been projected into the room. The analytic field was saturated with orphaned affect—dissociated desire, disavowed vulnerability, stylized shame. And I was left to metabolize it.

One afternoon, after Julian described a particularly degrading encounter, I found myself imagining what it felt like to be the other man in the scene. I wasn't fantasizing. I was *inhabiting* something—unbidden, uncanny. My reverie had been overtaken by a dissociated current that was not mine. I felt implicated, not violated—held inside something that couldn't be narrated yet. I came to understand this as more than countertransference. It was a **field effect**—Julian's unformulated erotic structure pressing into the contours of my perceptive self.

These moments clarified for me that reverie in dissociative erotic fields is not just a container for the patient's affect. It is a **receptor for aestheticized fragments**—longing without coherence, contact without continuity. The analyst becomes a kind of transitional object: not blank, but saturated. Not responsive, but receptive.

Eigen writes that in such states, the analyst may feel "strangely changed, not quite oneself." I began tracking these changes—not through interpretation, but through atmosphere. After sessions, I would jot words that floated up: "fog," "heat," "vacancy," "too much." These weren't notes for supervision. They were affective traces, part of the patient's erotic hologram, downloaded into my body.

Julian once asked—seemingly out of nowhere—"Do you ever feel like someone's watching you through your own eyes?" I paused. "Say more?" "It's just… sometimes I want something, and then I watch myself want it, and then it disappears."

That line illuminated the structure. He was not defending against desire. He was *witnessing himself from outside it*, unable to bear the simultaneity of wanting and being wanted. He needed distance—not to deny the erotic, but to survive its approach.

In these moments, the analyst's task is not to "bring the patient back." It is to remain near what is being expressed without form. To allow the erotic shimmer to exist in the room without grasping at coherence. To share the patient's self-exile.

My reverie became a kind of devotion—feeling for the patient, which could not yet be felt by them. I did not explain, decode, or direct. I remained. And over time, Julian's style softened. He began naming what he had previously only acted out. "I liked the way he looked at me," he said once. "But I also didn't want to be there."

The analyst in these treatments does not offer interpretation, but **embodied containment**. We bear the field until it becomes less frightening. We let the erotic live without collapsing it into desire or meaning. And sometimes, that bearing is enough.

Shame and the Temporality of Erotic Disavowal

In holographic erotic structures, shame is not an aftereffect. It is architectural. Not only does it contour how desire is allowed to emerge; it also shapes when it is permitted to arrive. In this terrain, the patient does not simply long and then feel ashamed. Instead, shame hovers **in anticipation**—structuring desire's possibility before it is even felt. This anticipatory shame distorts the temporal field. It renders the present unsafe, disqualifying affect before it can fully unfold.

Ava, a heterosexual woman in her late forties, came into treatment with a stated wish to "reclaim desire." Twice divorced, fluent in reflective language, she could speak about pleasure, even longing—but always at a distance. "I want to want," she said early in our work. "But I think I've forgotten how."

Her narratives of the past were vivid but curiously flat. She described lovers and encounters in detail, but without charge. The present, by contrast, was affectively muffled. Her dating life was perfunctory—organized around failure, not fantasy. "Desire feels like a job I'm bad at," she quipped.

I began to hear in Ava's voice not just inhibition but **temporal dissociation**. She wasn't cut off from desire as a drive—she was cut off from it as an unfolding experience. Pleasure had become something either pre-formulated or remembered from a safer distance. To feel in real time was too raw. Too dangerous.

Stern (1997) names this territory as "unformulated experience:" affect that was never mirrored, never integrated, and therefore never symbolized. But with Ava, what was striking was not simply what had gone unformulated—it was what had become *aestheticized*. She described erotic moments like they were curated artifacts. "I remember his mouth," she said once. "I can still picture it. But I don't remember what I felt." The erotic had been *archived*, not lived.

In this form, shame operates like a filter: not censoring what was felt, but preventing it from ever fully arriving. Ava once caught herself mid-thought and said, "Let's not name that—it'll disappear." She wasn't being evasive. She was protecting something too fragile to be spoken. The erotic shimmer would not survive exposure.

Julian offered another variation of this dynamic. His sexual fantasies were explicit, but emotionally suspended. He could describe being used, forgotten, humiliated—but always as if it had already happened to someone else. Even in the middle of a memory, he was narrating from after the effect had drained. It was as if he were describing desire's aftermath before it had begun. The erotic was narrated in **elegy**.

This is where time folds. The patient disowns the erotic by pre-empting its presence. Desire is rehearsed or remembered—but never embodied in the now. The shame is not about what they feel—it is about the risk of *still feeling*. Being in the erotic present would expose something unprotected.

With patients like Julian and Ava, interpretation often arrives too soon. The task is not to clarify, but to accompany—to sit with the patient in the slowed, muffled, glimmering field where desire almost speaks, where affect arrives in fragments. Where the erotic lives not in climax, but in hesitation.

Shame, here, is not an obstacle to desire. It is the condition that frames how desire is allowed to breathe. The analytic stance becomes not one of unveiling, but of **ethically reverent presence**. We do not push the effect forward. We remain near the moment that wants to form—and might never.

Another patient, Marcus, offered a more explicitly dissociative form of this temporal dislocation. A gay man in his late 20s, Marcus described himself as "sexually open but emotionally avoidant." He spoke of dozens of hookups with an easy, unaffected tone. When I asked how these experiences felt, his responses were consistent: "It was what it was." When I asked how he felt afterward, he said, "Fine. Or hungry. I usually just get food."

What Marcus couldn't articulate—but could perform—was a profound inability to inhabit the erotic in the presence of another. Intimacy was flattened. Contact was rendered transactional. But not out of numbness. Something more defensive was at work—an affective distance structured to maintain proximity without collapse.

He once described a hotel hookup with a man he didn't speak to. "He didn't even take off his shoes," Marcus said. "I think I liked that," I asked what he liked. He paused, then said: "That he didn't pretend it was anything more. I don't trust softness."

That line stayed with me: *I don't trust softness*. It named something deeper than avoidance. It named a refusal to be exposed to the vulnerability of being felt.

Marcus's fantasies revealed the structure more clearly. He preferred scenes of restraint, distance, and objectification—voyeurism, power play, being desired but untouched. "I like being seen more than being touched," he said. "Being touched means I have to feel something back."

Here again, temporality was shattered. The erotic was sculpted in such a way that the mutuality of feeling—the simultaneity of wanting and being wanted—was too much to bear. The hologram became a sanctuary: a space in which longing could be rehearsed without reciprocation.

Marcus's sessions were quiet, spare. He often folded into himself, covering his mouth or shielding his eyes when he spoke of anything emotionally alive. When I was too attuned, he'd shift the subject or poke at me. "You're very careful with me," he said once. "That scares me more than if you weren't."

I began to understand that tenderness, for Marcus, was a kind of threat. Erotic engagement structured around distance had become his way of protecting against exposure—not just physical, but psychic. As his analyst, I wasn't just witnessing this dynamic. I was drawn into it—hovering between too much and too little, seen but not addressed, felt but not named.

What I came to recognize was this: for patients like Marcus, the erotic hologram is not a barrier to connection—it is the structure through which connection becomes tolerable. Mutuality feels annihilating. Distance feels like contact. Presence must be carefully misaligned to be survivable.

When Marcus began seeing someone "kind of regularly," he was ambivalent. "It's not a relationship," he insisted. "We don't talk about feelings." I didn't challenge that. I stayed near it. He added, later, almost against his own will: "Sometimes I like it when he stays over. I pretend I'm asleep, but I know he's there."

This was not integration. But it was *contact*. A gesture toward presence. A shift in the field.

I didn't interpret. I said, "It sounds like something new is becoming possible."

He replied, "Maybe. Or maybe I'm just tired."

But he smiled. He knew I had heard what hadn't quite been said. And I knew he had risked letting me.

The Analyst's Double Position: Being Cast, Staying Human

In dissociative erotic structures, the analyst is not simply transferred upon—we are **cast**. We become characters in an aesthetic that precedes the analytic encounter. The patient doesn't only project; they **position** us. We are summoned into an unstable constellation of idealization, shame, longing, and avoidance. Sometimes, it is sacred. Sometimes as obscene. Sometimes, as both—often within the same hour.

With Julian, I was moved in and out of contradictory roles. There were weeks when I felt cast as the sanctified other—too pure to be touched by the material. "I don't want to ruin this," he'd say with a glance at the floor, changing the subject. Other times, I was the intruder. Once, when I asked gently about what a particular sexual scene left him feeling, he snapped: "I don't need you to psychoanalyze my dick."

I didn't respond. But I felt singed.

These weren't lapses in the frame. They were *the frame itself*. Julian was staging the erotic not through fantasy content, but through **relational choreography**. I wasn't outside it. I was inside the structure—shimmering, unstable, and affectively charged.

The analyst in such treatments becomes less an interpreter and more an instrument. We are playing. We resonate. And we absorb. My own body bore the effects of this over time. I noticed tightness in my chest before certain sessions. With Ava, a sense of breath-holding. With Marcus, a kind of post-session collapse. These were not ordinary countertransference affects. They were field reverberations—unspoken shards of erotic dissociation landing in my body.

I began to track my physical responses not as interference but as **clinical data**. Noticing when I leaned forward too gently. When I held my breath. When I felt erased. I wasn't looking for meaning. I was learning to **survive being misrecognized** without needing to correct the patient or reclaim my place.

At times, I could feel how delicate the choreography was. With Julian, a subtle shift in posture—a lean, a glance, a slight affective softening—could shift the entire field. In one session, I leaned in just slightly during a long silence. He flinched—barely—and said nothing. But the air thickened. The next week, he was distant. "Let's not go deep today," he said. "I'm tired."

It took time to learn that even nonverbal gestures of proximity were felt as rupture. Not because they were wrong, but because they were too close to something forbidden: the steady, caring, queerly present other. The one who might stay.

These moments forced me to reframe neutrality. The erotic isn't destabilized by analysis. It's destabilized by *presence*. By being near enough to be felt but not enacted. By being real, available, embodied—but not graspable.

In such fields, the analyst becomes a kind of **affective prism**—receiving, refracting, and metabolizing what the patient cannot yet hold. We are not blank screens. We are **somatic anchors**. Our task is not to purify the space but to remain intact inside the fragmentation.

This is what I mean by the analyst's double position. We are real, but used. Present, but misrecognized. We are called to **inhabit the contradiction**—to feel ourselves distorted and still remain.

This is not an interpretation. It is a kind of reverent waiting. A refusal to retaliate against miscasting. A willingness to remain human even when projected into positions that obscure us.

And we do so not because we are neutral—but because we are devoted to the possibility that something truer may one day enter the room.

Dissociation as Devotion—Toward a Clinical Poetics

The hologram, at first glance, reads as a defensive structure: an erotic architecture built to keep feeling out. But over time—if we stay near it—it reveals itself as something more nuanced. Not pathology. Not performance. **Devotion**. A structure the psyche has built not just to protect, but to honor something it once feared might be lost completely.

In the final year of our work, Julian began to speak less in clinical phrasing and more in hesitations. Where before he offered curated scripts—sexual scenes, emotional fragments, deadpan reflections—he now began to say things like, "I almost let myself feel something," or "It wasn't hot, but it was… something." His erotic narrative shifted not in content, but in **register**.

He told me once, "I used to think sex was the only place I existed. Now I'm not so sure that's true." It wasn't a revelation. It was a soft pivot. A shift in the air.

I said, "It sounds like something in you is starting to exist elsewhere."

He looked at me. "You stayed," he said. "That's what changed it."

What he meant was: *you stayed through the shimmer*. You didn't interpret me into wholeness. You didn't push the erotic into integration. You didn't leave when I disappeared. You bore my style.

This is where the analyst becomes something more than a reflective surface. We become **witnesses to aestheticized survival**. The erotic hasn't vanished. It's been layered and patterned. Fragmented in order to be preserved. And our task is to hear it *in that form*—in its partiality, its timing, its dissociation—not to force it into contact too soon.

I've come to think of these treatments as sites of poiesis. Not because we create the patient anew, but because we participate in an aesthetic field where survival takes the form of erotic style. We don't analyze the defenses—we accompany their tempo.

Derrida (1995) offers a language for this: the *undecidable*. An ethic of remaining in the opacity of what cannot yet be resolved. In these analytic encounters, the erotic field is often undecidable. To make meaning too quickly is to erase what is just beginning to form.

This is what makes the work so destabilizing—and so sacred. We are not helping the patient find "authentic" desire beneath the dissociation. We are staying long enough for the flicker to find a rhythm. For the erotic aesthetic to risk becoming **relational**.

This is not insight. It is resonance.

Structural Secrecy and the Erotic Architecture of Concealment

The *Madonna–whore–hologram* does not emerge ex nihilo. It is often the elaboration of a deeper condition: **secrecy as structure**. Especially in analytic work with queer men, I've found that the aestheticized form of erotic dissociation is not only defensive—it is developmental. It emerges in early relational and cultural environments where the erotic self is not simply shamed or ignored, but *pre-emptively concealed*.

Marcus, a patient I discussed earlier, recalled his first experience of sexual arousal at age ten. "It wasn't even sexual," he said. "It was just… a tingle in my spine and a warning bell at the same time. I knew right then—whatever this is, no one can know."

That moment wasn't a repression. It was a blueprint. Desire was marked not just by risk, but by a mandate to remain unspoken. From that point on, erotic feelings arrived paired with withdrawal. What Marcus eventually built was not an erotic life, but an **erotic aesthetic of disappearance**. To be seen was dangerous. To be felt was unbearable. So he became visible only through performance.

This kind of secrecy is not accidental. It is what Hans Loewald (1978a) might call a *developmental artifact*—a psychic arrangement formed not simply by inhibition, but by the absence of an other who could metabolize aliveness without recoil. Secrecy, in this light, is not the withholding of something known. It is the **preservation of something unformulatable**—an affect that would dissolve under the conditions available.

For queer patients, secrecy is often not a decision but a condition of being. Eve Sedgwick (1990) names the closet not as a location but as a **structural principle**—a way of managing exposure, desire, and relational risk through stylized concealment. The closet teaches a choreography: be visible, but not fully; speak, but through innuendo; desire, but never in real time. This becomes not only a relational strategy but a *style of selfhood*.

Adam Phillips (1996) writes that "secrets are the way we imagine we have a self." For patients formed in secrecy, the erotic becomes the core content of that imagined self—something too sacred, too shameful, or too charged to allow into the shared field. The secret becomes erotic not just for its content, but for its containment. The act of holding becomes the pleasure.

In these cases, the erotic is not disavowed because it is bad. It is encrypted because it is **unshareable without annihilation**.

What gets eroticized, then, is not just the other—but the *act of withholding*. The thrill of being almost seen. The repetition of being unreachable, even while touched. These are not failures of intimacy. They are its earliest form.

D. W. Winnicott (1965) offered the idea of the "true self" as something that must remain hidden to remain alive. Masud Khan (1983) extended this into the realm of secrecy—not as deception, but as a necessary "secret as potential space." He suggests that the secret—when protected rather than intruded upon—can become the basis for psychic coherence. In analytic work, this demands an extraordinary restraint: to know there is a secret and *not try to expose it*.

This helped me understand why Marcus and others like him eroticized partial contact. One patient, a corporate attorney in his forties, described only hooking up in public places: stairwells, gyms, alleys. "It's not the danger I like," he said. "It's the almost." He was not taking the risk. He was **sustaining erotic liveliness through curated concealment**.

Fairbairn (1944) and Guntrip (1969) both describe the schizoid dilemma of needing the object while fearing its approach. In these patients, I began to see that schizoid elements had been reworked—not into withdrawal, but into **stylization**. Erotic aesthetics became the solution to an old dilemma: how to be reached without collapsing. How to be seen without being devoured.

Foucault (1978) reminds us that secrecy is not always repressive. It can be *generative*. Power often functions not by silencing but by orchestrating forms of visibility. The queer subject learns this early. Erotic life becomes an exercise in **managing one's aperture**—revealing just enough to be wanted, never enough to be known.

The analyst, then, enters not just a private world, but a political aesthetic as well. One shaped by decades of learned opacity. In these treatments, our job is not to pry open the secret. It is to become the kind of presence around whom secrecy might one day soften.

Laing (1961) described secrecy as a "mode of existence." And for many queer patients, it is precisely that—a mode of living with feeling. A mode of being in the world with erotic life intact but unavailable.

Marcus once described a moment that illuminated this structure. He had been seeing someone casually—someone who began texting regularly, staying longer, lingering after sex. "One night," Marcus said, "he asked if he could shower here. It threw me."

He paused, then added, "I said yes, but I couldn't stay in the apartment. I went out to smoke, just to give him space. I felt like I was watching someone use my body from a distance."

It wasn't fear of the other—it was the **collapse of stylization**. A man showering in his apartment—too real, too continuous, too ordinary—pierced the erotic choreography Marcus relied on. The sexual could be held if it remained dissociated and discontinuous. But the **intimate residue of presence**? That was something else entirely.

I didn't interpret. I asked, "What was it that felt so different?"

He looked at the floor. "He wasn't disappearing."

And neither, it seemed, was Marcus.

Queer Embodiment and the Ethics of Being Seen

The analyst's body is never incidental. In erotic fields shaped by dissociation, the analyst's embodied presence often becomes one of the most charged dimensions of the work. And when that body is **queer**, its presence is not just perceptible—it is *structurally implicated*.

With Julian, my queerness was never named, but it was everywhere in the room. In his glances, in the flirtations he retracted, in the way he modulated his tone depending on my silences. I wasn't simply an analyst—I was a projected version of what he both feared and desired to become. Someone who had survived, or failed to survive, the erotic fracture he was still living inside.

When I responded with too much attunement, he would withdraw. When I held back, he would test me: *Don't pretend you don't know what I mean.* My queerness—my not-quite-spoken history—made me available in a way that also made me threatening. I wasn't part of the hologram, exactly. But my presence *animated it.*

This is the tension of queer embodiment in analytic work. We are too visible or too opaque, too similar or too unknowable. To queer patients, especially those structured by secrecy and stylization, the analyst's visibility carries both *promise and risk*. We are bodies that might recognize or bodies that might expose.

Harry Stack Sullivan (1953) emphasized the therapist's personality as the "basic tool" of the treatment—not to be revealed indiscriminately, but never truly absent. When the analyst is queer, this tool becomes ethically double-edged. Disclosure may be impossible. But erasure is no less dangerous. We must remain **tactile enough to be felt** without destabilizing the patient's defense.

Marcus would often refer obliquely to "guys like you." He didn't ask if I was gay. He created a field in which I had to be—without saying it. In one session, he said, "You seem like someone who wouldn't bother with stairwells." It wasn't a question. It was an invocation.

If I responded too warmly, he'd recoil. If I stayed neutral, he'd become sarcastic. He was watching how I inhabited my queerness. Could I be visible without shame? Present without stylization? Was I a collapsed version of his own future—or someone who had learned to survive softness?

To stay in the analytic seat in these moments was to inhabit a narrow channel—**neither embodying the patient's fantasy nor disavowing my difference**. It was to hold the erotic field with an integrity that did not collapse it.

Otto Rank (1936) might refer to this as the analyst's creative presence—not as a blank canvas, but as a responsive aesthetic force. We become instruments, not by being fully known, but by being *formally real*—attuned, ethical, and resistant to enactment.

These moments are not always reparative. They are felt **ruptures held in human form**. Julian once asked, "Were you always this comfortable in your skin?" I felt the tug to answer with honesty, solidarity, and biography. I didn't. I said, "It sounds like comfort is something you're thinking about."

He didn't answer. But something softened.

Buber (1970) writes that the *I–Thou* relationship requires real presence, not transparency. Mutuality doesn't mean sameness. It means being willing to show up as a bounded subject—alive, attentive, particular.

This is the queer ethic I try to hold as an analyst: *I will not abandon the field. But I will not colonize it either*. I will be here—not as your fantasy, not as your guide, but as a warm, visible other who stays even when cast badly.

And sometimes, that presence becomes the thing that reshapes the aesthetic. Not through insight. Through **witnessed coherence inside misrecognition**.

Conclusion: Reverence in the Field of Shimmer

To work within the *Madonna–whore–hologram* is to enter a terrain where erotic life has not failed but has been reorganized to survive contradiction. Here, the erotic is not absent—it is ritualized, withheld, delayed, refracted. The analyst is not only a recipient of projection; we are **drawn into an atmosphere** shaped by secrecy, shame, and premature aestheticization. What we find there is not pathology, but devotion.

These structures do not dissolve under interpretation. They do not integrate when named. Instead, they soften under **presence**—an analytic posture that neither demands coherence nor withdraws in the face of fragmentation.

The task is not to return the patient to some authentic erotic center. It is to accompany them through their *partially livable architecture*. To sit beside stylized distance without trying to bridge it. To feel desire shimmer and not reach for it.

What we offer is not resolution, but **resonance**. Not the fantasy of healing, but the actuality of shared opacity.

This is what I have come to understand as clinical reverence. A way of staying near the erotic—not to fix it, not to mirror it, but to witness it in its chosen form. To bear being miscast without retreating. To be a body in the field who does not require the patient to become more coherent than they can yet bear to be.

In these moments, what shifts is not the structure, but the solitude inside it. The patient remains stylized, yes. Fragmented, often. But no longer alone in the choreography.

And sometimes, that is enough.

Epilogue: A Flicker That Remains

Weeks after our final session, Julian sent me a short note. "Thanks for letting it be weird," he wrote. "I think that helped."

There was no elaboration. No summary of growth. Just the trace of a shared field—a shimmer we had both lived inside.

I find myself returning to that line: letting it be weird, not as a failure, but as an ethic. Perhaps the work is not always to render the erotic legible, but to remain with its illegibility long enough that something human begins to stir. A flicker. A fragment. A gesture toward presence.

In that sense, the hologram never resolves. It fades and returns, shifts and reconstitutes. And if we're lucky—if we are careful—it begins to carry less loneliness.

6 The Dialectic of Coherence and Containment

Ferenczi's Legacy and the Ethics of Listening

This chapter revisits Sándor Ferenczi's clinical legacy through the dialectic of coherence and containment. Coherence refers to the drive to symbolize, narrate, and make meaning; containment refers to the capacity to hold affective states that have not yet been integrated. Drawing from relational psychoanalysis, this chapter argues that therapeutic action lies in the analyst's modulation of these forces—especially in the context of trauma, dissociation, and enactment. Engaging theorists including Loewald, Orange, Benjamin, Harris, and Laplanche, it highlights how the ethics of listening, countertransference pressure, and analytic timing shape the capacity for symbolization. Clinical vignettes illustrate how disruptions in this dialectic produce impasses and how repair often depends not on interpretation alone but on the analyst's disciplined presence. The framework has implications for working with fragmented experience and for training analysts to track the relational field without prematurely imposing coherence.

Introduction: Ferenczi after Interpretation

Few texts in the psychoanalytic canon are as hauntingly unfinished as Ferenczi's 1933 "Confusion of Tongues." More an open wound than a theoretical treatise, it offers a vision of trauma not only as a violent intrusion but as *misattunement in language*. The betrayal Ferenczi describes is twofold: the child's gestures of tenderness are not only misread but answered in the register of adult passion, producing not just psychic fragmentation, but a collapse in the possibility of shared meaning. The seduction is epistemic as much as it is physical—an annihilation of the child's own capacity to name their experience.

Contemporary psychoanalytic theorists have returned to Ferenczi's work with reverence and anxiety. Writers such as Judith Dupont, Arnold Rachman, Jay Frankel, and others have emphasized his early recognition of trauma's dissociative impact and his revolutionary stance on mutuality, countertransference, and analytic ethics. At the same time, his work has been criticized for its experimental excesses, including his practice of mutual analysis. But beneath these clinical debates lies a deeper contribution: Ferenczi's insistence that the

DOI: 10.4324/9781003715283-9

analyst must bear witness not only to the content of trauma, but to the *structural conditions under which psychic life becomes narratable.*

This chapter proposes that Ferenczi's clinical vision can be reframed through a contemporary dialectic between **coherence** and **containment**. Rather than opposing techniques or theoretical allegiances, these functions are mutually constitutive poles of analytic action—each necessary for therapeutic transformation, and each potentially disruptive when dislocated from the other. In this formulation, coherence refers to the drive for meaning, symbolization, and narrative; containment refers to the capacity to hold affect and dissociation without rushing toward interpretation. Their tension is not only technical, but ethical.

I argue that this dialectic lies at the heart of Ferenczi's late work, offering a framework for understanding clinical impasses, enactments, and the analyst's emotional posture. Drawing on theorists including Loewald, Benjamin, Orange, Harris, Laplanche, and Bion, I situate coherence and containment within contemporary debates on trauma, symbolization, and relational authority. Through clinical vignettes and micro-process reflections, I show how the analyst's disciplined modulation of this dialectic can restore the conditions for meaning where they have collapsed.

What follows is organized into three parts. One section explores the theoretical and developmental interweaving of coherence and containment. Another section focuses on coherence as both healing and potentially seductive. A later section reframes containment as a generative clinical stance. An additional section traces enactments and dialectical rupture. An ending section offers clinical material, and the final sections reflect on temporality, witnessing, and the ethical demands of analytic listening.

While this chapter is grounded in clinical theory, it is also informed by a relational-constructivist view of psychoanalysis (Hoffman, 1998; Orange, 1995), in which the analyst's stance and participation shape what becomes thinkable. Clinical material is drawn from a contemporary relational practice, with attention to countertransference, affective pacing, and symbolization. The goal is not to offer a technical procedure, but to illuminate how the dialectic of coherence and containment emerges moment to moment in the intersubjective field.

A Dialectic Emerges: From Ferenczi to the Present

Ferenczi's contribution to psychoanalysis is often situated in his clinical innovations: the analyst's use of tenderness, countertransference transparency, and the technical implications of trauma-induced dissociation. But Ferenczi was also among the first to insist that interpretation itself could be retraumatizing—that to offer meaning prematurely, or from the wrong register, could re-enact the very confusion the patient originally suffered.

This concern reappears throughout relational and intersubjective theory. Hans Loewald (1978a) envisioned the psyche as a dynamic field in which unintegrated experience is gradually transformed into coherent symbolic form—a process that depends on the internalization of attuned relational functions. Coherence, in Loewald's account, is not a given but a developmental product, contingent upon the availability of containing others who can metabolize raw experience without foreclosing its meaning too soon.

Jessica Benjamin (1990, 1998) reframes this process through the lens of recognition. To be recognized, for Benjamin, is to have one's subjectivity affirmed without appropriation. The analyst must resist the pull to explain or understand the patient *too well*—a form of epistemic mastery that reproduces the asymmetries of early misattunement. In this sense, premature coherence becomes a form of seduction, echoing the adult's appropriation of the child's tenderness that Ferenczi so vividly described.

Donna Orange (1995, 2010) centers the analyst's capacity for emotional understanding, arguing that containment without empathic attunement becomes sterile, while coherence without ethical humility becomes intrusive. Her work reminds us that the patient's affective idiom must be *received* before it is *interpreted*—and that this receiving is not passive, but a deeply embodied relational labor.

Adrienne Harris (2009) adds to this by situating analytic authority within broader power structures. Her account of *relational discipline* insists that the analyst must hold their authority lightly, aware that even silence or attunement may be experienced as regulation or erasure. The patient's protest—against being explained, soothed, or held without engagement—becomes a clue to the fragile equilibrium between coherence and containment.

Finally, Jean Laplanche's (1999) theory of the *enigmatic signifier* crystallizes the core of the confusion Ferenczi identified. The adult's unconscious, sedimented in language and gesture, implants meanings in the child's psyche that the child is not developmentally equipped to decode. The resulting psychic pressure is not only affective but hermeneutic: a drive to translate the untranslatable, to render coherent what was never meant for the child's understanding. Here, the trauma lies in meaning itself—too much, too soon, too foreign. Sometimes, dissociative stillness becomes a form of ethical refusal: a resistance to the violence of premature meaning when the world's grammar has not yet earned the right to name the self.

In all of these accounts, we find a shared thread: the analyst's task is not to interpret or contain in isolation, but to inhabit a relational field in which the patient's experience may become sayable without being forced to say.

Misattunement as Structural Trauma

The theoretical grounding laid above positions us to deepen one core idea: that misattunement is not simply a momentary rupture but a sustained condition—a *structural trauma* that forecloses the possibility of coherence. One section explores how Ferenczi's ideas anticipated this framing and how later theorists have built on it.

Ferenczi's account of trauma in *Confusion of Tongues* goes beyond any singular event of seduction or betrayal. What he illuminates, often only implicitly, is that trauma also arises from the chronic failure of the adult to match the child's mode of communication. The parent does not simply abuse; they *misattune*, repeatedly and structurally, speaking the wrong language, offering the wrong kind of presence, or foreclosing meaning before it can emerge. This misattunement—especially when cloaked in care—generates not just affective injury, but a deep fracture in the child's sense of relational safety and symbolic authorship. In this way, Ferenczi can be understood as an early theorist of what later writers would call **structural trauma**: a form of psychic injury not tied to a singular event, but to the *patterned invalidation* of meaning, experience, and emerging selfhood.

Robert Stolorow (2007) provides a contemporary rendering of this principle. In his concept of **emotional trauma as contextually embedded**, Stolorow argues that trauma is not reducible to content alone but occurs when affective experience is met with absence, dismissal, or distortion by the caregiver. In such cases, the affect cannot be regulated intersubjectively; it cannot be "held" in the relational field. It remains unformulated, dissociated, or prematurely regulated by the child's own compensatory mechanisms—intellectualization, submission, withdrawal. In this light, Ferenczi's concern with the analyst's tone, pacing, and elasticity may be read as an early attempt to address what Stolorow later calls *the failure of attunement to the context of the patient's affective life*.

Similarly, Peter Fonagy's work on **epistemic trust** intersects closely with Ferenczi's concerns. Fonagy and colleagues (Fonagy et al., 2015) describe how the capacity to learn from others—to treat the communications of others as trustworthy and relevant—is built developmentally through interactions in which emotional experience is mirrored *accurately, contingently, and marked as belonging to the child*. When caregivers routinely override or misattribute the child's inner states, epistemic trust collapses. The result is not merely interpersonal mistrust, but a defensive structure organized around the *avoidance of new meaning*. In these individuals, the analyst's efforts to offer coherence may be met with suspicion, dread, or psychic retreat—not because the interpretation is wrong, but because the conditions of trust necessary to receive it have not been established.

This helps explain the common clinical picture in which a patient's **fragmentation is not in response to trauma per se**, but in response to the analytic encounter itself. The therapist's attempt to name experience, however tentatively, may be experienced as a repetition of structural misattunement: another well-intentioned adult who speaks in the wrong register, who wants too much too fast, who listens with the intention to understand rather than the willingness to be changed. These patients often inhabit what Bromberg (1998) calls *multiple self-states* that resist integration, precisely because integration feels like colonization.

In this context, containment and coherence must be rethought not as techniques, but as **conditions of epistemic restoration**. The analyst must create an environment in which the patient's meaning can begin to feel narratable—not through the force of interpretation, but through a form of listening that attunes not only to what is said, but to *how saying itself has been structured by past violation*. As Adrienne Harris (2009) notes, trauma often results in *a compromised capacity to symbolize without dissociation*. The analytic task is not to push the patient toward coherence but to track how coherence itself has become threatening and to offer containment that allows coherence to become safe again.

In this way, Ferenczi's language of "tongues" becomes a prescient metaphor for epistemic safety. The goal is not to translate the patient, but to meet them in their idiom, to become literate in the form their suffering has taken. Only from there can coherence become something other than seduction—something co-authored, symbolically authentic, and affectively survivable.

From Holding to Meaning: The Developmental Roots of the Dialectic

If misattunement marks a failure of relational rhythm, how do coherence and containment emerge developmentally in their optimal form? Early dyadic processes—from mother–infant interaction to affect attunement—show how these functions are co-constructed from the beginning.

Although coherence and containment may appear as technical choices within the clinical hour—to interpret or to hold, to speak or to remain silent—their roots lie deep within the earliest relational matrices of infancy. They are not merely interventions, but developmental capacities: forged in the crucible of the caregiver–infant relationship, they emerge together, each scaffolding the other. This interdependency is often obscured in discussions of analytic technique, which often polarize holding and interpretation. But to understand their dialectic force clinically, one must first recognize them as **co-emergent developmental functions**.

Infant observation studies, such as those by Beatrice Beebe and colleagues (1997), demonstrate that infants seek not just soothing but *patterned coherence* in the caregiver's responses. The infant looks for rhythms, for contingent mirroring, for the return of affect in recognizable form. In this view, containment is not simply the capacity to absorb distress, but to do so in a way that renders experience *narratable over time*. When the mother's gaze, voice, and touch reflect back the infant's internal state in a modulated, marked, and contingent fashion, the infant begins to develop an implicit sense of coherence—a felt continuity of self-in-experience.

In object relations theory, this principle has long been articulated through metaphor. Winnicott's (1965) notion of the **holding environment** describes a maternal function that allows the infant to sustain being without collapse. But for Winnicott, this environment does not simply shelter; it is the very precondition for symbol formation. Without holding, the infant cannot play. Without play, the infant cannot discover a mind of its own. Containment, then, is what allows coherence to take symbolic form. It is not prior to narrative—it is the breathing room within which narrative becomes possible.

Wilfred Bion, in his elaboration of the alpha function, adds another layer. The mother's containment allows the infant's beta elements—raw, unprocessed emotional data—to be digested into forms the infant can begin to symbolize. The translation of chaos into nascent coherence begins in this interpersonal matrix. In adult analytic work, the analyst recapitulates this function by receiving the patient's dissociated material not only silently but **transformationally**. Coherence becomes possible when containment is not just passive, but metabolizing—when the analyst can feel without flooding and think without foreclosing.

Contemporary affect theory has similarly emphasized the *co-regulatory function* of narrative and presence. Daniel Stern's (1985) work on affect attunement shows that the infant is not simply calmed by the parent's presence; they are developmentally shaped by the parent's **modulated joining** of their inner state. This joining is never identical—the parent does not mirror exactly, but offers an emotionally legible version of the child's distress. In this way, containment is not blank; it is *symbolically generative*. It teaches the child not just that they can be held, but that their inner states can become *knowable* and *known* through relationship.

What emerges from these converging perspectives is a portrait of coherence and containment as **inseparable in early development**, though often disaggregated in clinical theory. The infant does not first get held and then get interpreted. Rather, they are held *in such a way* that their experience gradually becomes coherent. The mother does not tell the child what the child feels, but she feels it with them in a form that makes sense. The analyst's task is not so different. When we hold without imposing coherence, we re-enact a failed early possibility. When we interpret without containment, we risk repeating the violence of meaning unearned.

Ferenczi did not have the language of affect regulation or developmental neuroscience, but his sensitivity to the psychic injury caused by misattunement placed him far ahead of his time. His insistence that the analyst attend not only to what is said but to how it is heard, not only to what the patient feels but to what the analyst's response does to that feeling, marks the beginning of a dialectical ethic in psychoanalysis. Coherence and containment are not theoretical options. They are relationally scaffolded capacities whose clinical rhythm must be rediscovered anew with every patient. And when those rhythms are profoundly absent or violated, what may look like psychic collapse may in fact represent an **ethical refusal**—a quiet stand against the imposition of meaning that has not been earned.

Coherence: The Seduction of Sense and the Pressure to Narrate

If containment refers to the capacity to hold affective experience without premature foreclosure, coherence refers to the psychic demand to make meaning from the held material. Ferenczi's clinical sensitivity to the child's subjugation to adult desire did not merely hinge on the violation of bodily boundaries. It also implicated the *imposed coherence* of adult meaning. In his "Confusion of Tongues" thesis, Ferenczi articulated how the adult misreads the child's tender gestures through the language of passion, not only acting upon the child's body but colonizing the child's meaning-making apparatus with an alien grammar (Ferenczi, 1933). The trauma, then, is not only that of violent intrusion, but of a prematurely enforced narrative—a collapse of psychic sovereignty beneath the seduction of imposed sense.

Later theorists have addressed this tension in different ways. Hans Loewald (1978c) viewed psychic integration as a developmental task rooted in the internalization of parental functions, emphasizing that the movement from unformed affect to symbolized experience depends upon the holding structures of the ego. For Loewald, coherence is not given, but achieved: a product of symbolization rooted in the relationship between self and object. In this sense, Ferenczi's concern anticipates Loewald's model—in the case of traumatic seduction, the parent is not facilitating symbol formation but instead imposing a pseudo-symbolic overlay, one that invalidates the child's nascent experiential categories.

Jessica Benjamin (1990, 1998) adds that recognition—the experience of being seen without distortion—is essential to the formation of coherent subjectivity. The trauma of misrecognition, as Ferenczi foreshadowed, is not merely a failure of empathy but a collapse in the reflective function of the other. The child is not mirrored, but mirrored *wrongly*—seen through the lens of adult sexuality, denied the language of tenderness. Thus, the coherence offered by the adult is not felt as authentic but as invasive, driving a wedge between experience and expression.

This dynamic is central to what Donna Orange (1995) has called *emotional understanding*. For Orange, the clinical task is to support the patient's emergent coherence by attuning to their idiomatic emotional language without erasing its ambiguity. Emotional coherence is not the product of intellectual interpretation, but of a shared process of meaning-making in which the patient's experience is held long enough to find its form. This resonates deeply with Ferenczi's emphasis on *tact*, *elasticity*, and the analyst's willingness to participate in a relational field where coherence must be earned rather than assumed.

Coherence, then, is not a neutral good. It is both a developmental necessity and a site of danger. As Laplanche (1999) warns, interpretation is always haunted by the risk of *re-seduction*: the imposition of coherence from the position of the supposed knowing other. The enigmatic signifiers of the adult world—those unprocessed residues of the adult's unconscious—are deposited into the child's psyche, forcing translation before there is any native capacity to metabolize their content. The result is not symbolic thought, but symbolic foreclosure disguised as comprehension.

In the clinical setting, this history is often re-enacted. Patients arrive in states of fragmentation, seeking coherence—but not at any cost. They seek to be held in the *possibility* of meaning without being forced to prematurely adopt one. The analyst, too, is vulnerable: to the pull of explanation, the illusion of clarity, the transference invitation to "make sense of me." The dialectic of coherence and containment thus reasserts itself: interpretation must emerge from within containment, not as a substitute for it. To narrate too soon is to echo the original trauma—to confuse the language of passion for the language of tenderness once again.

Clinical Vignette: "Isabelle" and the Violence of Interpretation

Isabelle, a woman in her early forties, came to treatment following what she described as an "emotional disappearance." After a series of relational ruptures—a divorce, a loss of spiritual community, the death of a beloved aunt—she found herself unable to speak about what she was feeling. "I used to be able to put things into words," she told me early on, "but now language just feels like a form of betrayal."

In our initial sessions, Isabelle often sat quietly, eyes closed, sometimes rocking gently. When she spoke, her words were halting and elliptical. Images surfaced—a moth caught in a lampshade, a warm wind that turns suddenly cold—but they came unanchored from narrative. She sometimes apologized: "This probably doesn't make sense." But when I tried to respond with gentle interpretations, offering potential emotional threads or linking present experience to earlier themes, she would flinch. "No — that's not what I mean. You're making it tidy."

In supervision, I found myself frustrated and anxious. I had the sense that she needed help symbolizing her experience, and yet every attempt to do so was experienced as a coercion. Her images were evocative but refused translation. I began to recognize the particular valence of her protest: she did not simply fear being misunderstood, but being *over-understood*—consumed by a meaning she had not chosen.

As our work unfolded, a more direct account of early trauma emerged. Her mother, a psychoanalyst, had often offered running commentary on Isabelle's emotional states. "She would tell me what I was feeling," Isabelle recalled, "before I even knew it myself. I learned to smile and say thank you for interpretations that made me feel hollow inside." The adult world had offered her coherence, but not containment. Narrative arrived as an alien graft—an interpretation imposed in the absence of being held.

In the transference, I had become that knowing mother. Even my most tentative interventions were experienced as appropriations. It became clear that what Isabelle needed first was *containment without interpretation*. I began to speak less. I allowed long silences to remain unfilled. When she looked at me with the beginnings of fear or protest, I would sometimes say softly, "I'm here. We don't have to make it make sense yet."

Gradually, the room became a place where her internal fragments could drift, reconfigure, and find new associations—on her terms. She began to write poems between sessions. She once brought in a line: "The meaning lives behind the curtain, waiting for the breath to pull it aside." In time, Isabelle began to reach for coherence herself—not to please me, not to fend off chaos, but as an act of creative agency. When she did, her stories retained their texture and strangeness. She allowed me to reflect back tentative meanings, but now we co-constructed them, shaping coherence from within containment rather than imposing it from without.

Clinical Vignette: "Jared" and the Ache for Meaning

Jared, a 31-year-old man working in publishing, entered treatment after a series of panic attacks disrupted his capacity to function at work. He described himself as "introspective to a fault," and his intake history was filled with the language of self-analysis: "I intellectualize too much," "I'm probably repressing something," "I tend to overthink my own childhood."

Yet in session, Jared spoke in waves—urgent, then suddenly incoherent. He would narrate events clearly for five minutes and then lose his thread, backtrack, or contradict himself. "I know I'm not making sense," he'd mutter, frustration mounting. I initially responded with steady containment—listening quietly, offering minimal validation: "It's okay not to make sense right now." My hope was to create space for a less pressured, more emotionally grounded experience of being heard.

But over the following weeks, Jared grew agitated. "I feel like I'm falling apart in here," he snapped one day. "You just sit there like you're watching a storm, waiting for it to pass. I don't need a lifeguard. I need a translator."

That line stayed with me. He didn't want to simply be held—he wanted *witnessing through meaning*. Jared had grown up with parents who were well-meaning but emotionally erratic. His mother cycled between effusive intimacy and chilling withdrawal; his father, an emotionally distant academic, responded to Jared's distress by handing him books. "I had to put myself together," he said. "I needed coherence — I made myself into a story just to survive."

In the transference, my withholding interpretations had not registered as attunement but as absence—another adult turning inward instead of meeting him. My attempt at containment had inadvertently mirrored the chilly space of his father's silence, confirming Jared's sense that affect had no communicable form. I realized that my own caution—my wish to avoid imposing coherence as violence—had caused me to forget that *coherence can also be care*.

In subsequent sessions, I began to offer gentle meaning-making efforts. I reflected on shifts in his emotional tone. I linked his sense of fragmentation to the sudden loss of structure in a recent romantic breakup. I was careful not to explain to him, but to offer threads—linguistic holding environments—that might become shared. He softened. "That helps," he whispered once. "Even if it's not quite right, it helps to have a frame."

Over time, Jared and I developed a rhythm in which he could reject or reshape my formulations without feeling engulfed by them. The frame held, but it bent with him. Coherence emerged not as totalization but as the promise of a shared grammar—one built slowly, reciprocally, through presence and language alike.

Containment: Holding the Unnarrated without Imposing Form

If coherence speaks to the psychic demand for intelligibility, containment refers to the analyst's capacity to *receive what cannot yet be spoken*. Ferenczi's late work turned increasingly toward this function. In *Confusion of Tongues*, he described not only the betrayal of seduction but also the rupture of the relational envelope—the absence of a protective frame in which the child's experience could unfold safely. His experiments with mutual analysis and his emphasis on the analyst's tenderness were less a turn toward permissiveness than an effort to establish the *conditions for containment* that might precede symbolic repair.

The idea of containment as a primary analytic function finds its most structured elaboration in Bion's (1962) concept of the **alpha function**—the mind's capacity to metabolize raw, unprocessed experience. When the infant projects overwhelming feelings into the mother, it is the mother's *reverie*, her capacity to absorb and transform them, that allows the infant to gradually develop a mind of its own. In analysis, this maternal function is re-enacted: the analyst contains not only the patient's affects but the fragments of thought, image, and drive that cannot yet be integrated into a coherent ego structure. To contain is to hold without interpretation—to receive the unnamable without reflexively pressing it into form.

But containment, like coherence, is not morally neutral. As Michael Eigen (1986) reminds us, containment may border on deadness if it does not vibrate with the textures of presence. "Containment without passion becomes a kind of crypt," he writes—a hollow frame. Eigen's work offers a necessary corrective to overly structural understandings of containment: he emphasizes its *aesthetic and affective dimensions*. To contain another's experience is not merely to survive it, but to be touched by it without flooding or collapse. Containment, in this view, is not just an envelope—it is a resonant skin.

Thomas Ogden (1994) carries this further in his conception of the **analytic third**: containment occurs not only in the analyst's mind but in the co-created intersubjective field. It is not the analyst alone who contains, but the analytic relationship that becomes a space where psychic fragments can be dreamed into being. Ferenczi's experiments with countertransference self-disclosure were early efforts to activate this field, to refuse the dead objectivity of the neutral analyst and instead offer an enlivened presence capable of holding dissociated experience. In this, Ferenczi anticipated Ogden's call for *aesthetic reciprocity* in containment—a jointly authored space where the unknown may emerge and take form.

Donna Orange (2010) reframes containment in ethical terms. For her, the analyst's primary task is **empathic responsibility**—a disciplined attunement to the patient's unique subjectivity, particularly in the wake of trauma. Orange warns against the instrumentalization of containment: if it becomes a technique, it risks reproducing the very dehumanization it seeks to remedy. True containment, she argues, is *witnessing without colonization*. It is the willingness to be changed by what the other brings—to hold it without digesting it for them. Here we see a profound resonance with Ferenczi's ethic of tenderness: not an absence of boundaries, but a refusal to dominate the terms of experience. Shapiro (2020) similarly argues that in work with traumatized patients, the analyst's capacity to tolerate unformulated states without moving prematurely into coherence is often the decisive factor in preserving the therapeutic frame.

Adrienne Harris (2009) brings yet another dimension, locating containment within power dynamics and relational asymmetries. For Harris, containment must always contend with the analyst's structural authority—the potential to soothe or silence, to witness or overwrite. In this sense, containment is not merely a function but a stance: a refusal to enact the omnipotence so often projected onto the analyst. In the clinical dialectic, containment holds the line against the fantasy of coherence as a cure. It insists that the analyst not complete the patient's sentence too quickly—not tidy the mess that may need, for a time, to remain messy.

Together, these perspectives underscore containment's complexity: it is not a passive holding, but an active, receptive discipline. It is a mode of being-with that refuses both seduction and abandonment. In Ferenczi's terms, it is the restoration of a language of tenderness, where what has been violated can be remet with care. In the dialectic with coherence, containment does not resist meaning—it *makes meaning possible* by first granting experience the time and space to unfurl in its own tempo. Without containment, coherence becomes coercive. Without coherence, containment becomes mute. It is in their oscillation—their attuned dialectic—that therapeutic transformation unfolds.

The Dialectic of Coherence and Containment: Clinical Impasses and Relational Repair

While coherence and containment can be described discretely, they rarely operate in isolation. Their dynamic tension forms the ground of the analytic process, especially in work with patients whose early relational environments were shaped by disavowal, seduction, or psychic overwhelm. Ferenczi's late clinical vision, radical for its time, presaged this dialectical complexity. He saw that the analyst's task is not to interpret *or* to hold but to engage in a responsive, ethically attuned dance between the two, allowing meaning to unfold without rushing or retreating from it.

When this balance collapses, clinical impasses often emerge. If the analyst privileges **coherence without containment**, the patient may feel exposed, intruded upon, or subtly coerced into meaning structures that do not yet feel safe. This may appear in patients like Isabelle, who reject interpretations not because they are wrong, but because they come too soon—before the psychic soil has been tilled for their planting. These patients often protest not the content of the interpretation, but its *timing*, its affective pressure, its implicit demand that the self become legible before it feels held.

Conversely, when the analyst leans too far into **containment without coherence**, patients may experience the treatment as floating, unmoored. Jared's reaction—"I don't need a lifeguard, I need a translator"—reflects this disorientation. In these moments, the analyst's silence, however well-intentioned, risks becoming a mirror of early parental absence: the withholding of meaning as a form of disconnection. The patient's emergent meanings are not simply held—they are left to dissipate, unacknowledged, in the analytic ether. Containment without the risk of coherence can devolve into what Ogden (2005c) called *non-responsiveness masked as neutrality*.

The dialectic, then, requires a form of **attuned instability**. It demands that the analyst oscillate—sometimes within the same session—between making room and making sense. In this, the analyst becomes both participant and witness, both container and meaning-maker. This echoes Thomas Ogden's (1994) view of the *analytic third* as a co-created psychic space where experience can be simultaneously *felt* and *thought*, *held* and *named*. Ferenczi's work prefigures this—especially in his willingness to step into the patient's affective world, even at the cost of analytic orthodoxy.

Michael Eigen (2004) offers a resonant metaphor here: he describes containment as "thickening the present," allowing the moment to gain depth and texture without prematurely evacuating it into narrative. Coherence, then, becomes an emergent property—a *felt sense* that arises from sustained presence, rather than a product imposed from without. In this model, interpretation is not an act of closure but of *co-sensing*—a shared attempt to metabolize what is arising.

This dialectic also reframes the transference-countertransference matrix. Patients often unconsciously pressure analysts toward one pole or the other. Some seduce the analyst into omniscient coherence—pulling for explanation, symbolization, or rescue via meaning. Others evoke a defensive containment—saturating the analytic field with affect while resisting integration. In either case, the analyst's capacity to tolerate *the pressure to fix*—to resist becoming either interpreter or inert container—becomes the hinge upon which therapeutic possibility rests.

Moreover, the dialectic offers a structural frame for understanding certain enactments. For example, when the analyst prematurely interprets a dissociated affect, it may not be the content but the *collapse of containment* that is retraumatizing. Or when the analyst remains silent during a moment saturated with emergent meaning, it may not be the withholding itself but the *loss of coherence* that evokes abandonment. Understanding these missteps not as technical failures but as ruptures in the coherence-containment matrix allows for more nuanced repair.

Ultimately, the analyst must cultivate a **dialectical posture**: one that neither seeks to stabilize the patient too quickly through imposed meaning nor avoids the tension of naming altogether. This requires what Harris (2009) calls *relational discipline*: a willingness to risk, to wait, to err, and to mend—all in the service of a shared language that arises not from the analyst's authority, but from the intersubjective space they co-create with the patient.

In returning to Ferenczi with this lens, we do not merely honor his radical tenderness—we extend it. We see that his concern with misattunement was not only about the confusion of affective languages, but about the failure of analytic function when it becomes unidimensional. He reminds us that healing takes place not at the poles of sense or holding, but in their ongoing interplay—where the psyche learns, again, to mean what it feels and feel what it means.

Enactments and Countertransference Pressure in the Coherence–Containment Dialectic

The coherence–containment dialectic is not only a developmental frame or a technique of listening. It is also a **structure of tension** within the analyst's own mind and body—one that surfaces most vividly in moments of countertransference pressure and analytic enactment. These are not merely slips in neutrality, but often the most affectively saturated expressions of where the analyst has lost the dialectical balance—pulled too far into coherence or too long into containment, seduced by knowing or paralyzed by care.

Enactments are frequently preceded by an unformulated pressure within the dyad: a feeling that something must be done, something must be said, something is being asked of the analyst but cannot be named. In these moments, the dialectic begins to tilt. The analyst may feel the need to rescue the patient from confusion through insight, a pressure toward premature coherence—often rationalized as therapeutic clarity. Or they may feel themselves sliding into wordless absorption, holding more and more affect without symbolic intervention, fearing that any interpretation will be experienced as intrusion. Both represent failures in the analyst's **internal dialectic**, where presence and thought, containment and meaning, lose their fluidity.

Ferenczi's legacy is particularly useful here. His own enactments—including the controversial mutual analysis—were arguably less evidence of personal instability than of an unregulated countertransference pull: a profound sensitivity to the patient's unmet need coupled with an insufficiently metabolized analytic frame. He was pulled toward radical forms of containment and identification, but at the cost of losing symbolic differentiation. His technical failures, then, can be read as the cost of holding too much without symbolic re-entry—a failure to oscillate back into coherence.

Contemporary relational theorists such as Philip Bromberg (2006) and Irwin Hoffman (1998) have emphasized that enactments often represent **intersubjective co-creations** rather than technical errors. They emerge when something is being enacted that cannot yet be mentalized—often because the analyst has unconsciously taken up a role the patient requires, resists, or both. In this view, countertransference is not noise but data: a clue to where the dialectic has collapsed and where repair must begin. The analyst may realize, for instance, that their silence has ceased to be holding and has become withdrawal—or that their interpretive reach has subtly silenced the patient's affective authority. As Stern (2015) notes, enactments often crystallize the implicit tension between the analyst's containing function and the patient's drive toward coherence, emerging as moments of shared, affectively saturated meaning that cannot yet be articulated.

At these crossroads, the temptation is toward one-sided solutions: to interpret the enactment as a return to insight (coherence) or to retreat into neutrality and empathy (containment). But what is required instead is **re-entry into dialectical tension**—to sustain thought without abandoning affect, and to speak without severing contact. These moments demand what Harris (2009) calls *relational discipline*—the analyst's capacity to stay in the heat of psychic intensity without becoming either the expert or the empathic void.

In supervision, such enactments often show up as statements like: "I didn't know what to say," or "Whatever I said felt like too much." These are signs not of failure, but of dialectical overload—the breakdown of the analyst's internal balance between containing presence and interpretive activity. Training, in this light, becomes not only about learning to interpret or to hold, but learning to bear the **oscillation**—to stay near the zone of dialectical ambiguity where the most transformative work occurs.

Moreover, recognizing enactments through this lens reframes repair. Rather than apologizing for interpretation or compensating with affective validation, the analyst can name the oscillation itself: "It felt like I was trying too hard to make this make sense. I wonder if that felt distancing." Or, conversely: "I've been so careful not to overwhelm you that I may have left you too alone with what you're carrying." These metacommunications do more than explain. They restore the analytic third—that shared space in which thinking and feeling can be rejoined.

Through this lens, enactments become part of the dialectic, not interruptions of it. They show where the system tilts, where the analyst's own capacity to hold and symbolize has narrowed, and where the patient is pulling—often urgently, if unconsciously—for the analyst to survive a relational position that once failed them. Enactments, then, are not merely ruptures. They are invitations to return to the field of tension where coherence and containment can be re-stitched—not through mastery, but through responsiveness and renewed dialectical presence.

Clinical Vignette: "Ethan" and the Demand to Stay Outside

Ethan, a 46-year-old attorney, came to treatment reluctantly, referred by a colleague who had noticed Ethan's increasing withdrawal and "emotional volatility at work." During our initial meetings, Ethan was punctual, articulate, and poised. He spoke fluently and insightfully about his family, his work, and even his "tendency to over-control everything." He spoke of emotional experience the way a physicist might speak of heat: with clarity, but at a distance.

While Ethan acknowledged that he was "not very connected to feelings," he was also quick to reassure me that he didn't expect therapy to fix that. "I'm here to be practical," he said. "I want better tools for managing stress — not to unearth repressed memories or get into some emotional soup."

In early sessions, I responded with careful attention and quiet presence, inviting him to linger in pauses, to notice shifts in tone, or to allow certain moments to remain unformulated. But these efforts at containment—at simply being with him—were met with irritation. "I feel like you're waiting for me to say something I don't have access to," he said one day. "Can't we just talk like two adults?" I found myself feeling subtly rebuked for creating what I imagined to be a space of safety. But to Ethan, that space was not safe—it was vague, unstructured, even threatening.

Over time, I began to appreciate that Ethan was not resisting affect; he was resisting *being held* in a way that implied something unspoken needed tending. His lifelong strategy had been coherence without containment—staying in control of his narrative, mastering language, shaping himself into a knowable, legible self. My efforts to offer containment, however minimal, disrupted his strategy. Where I hoped to offer room, he experienced a demand. My silence was not neutral—it was saturated with implication. The frame itself had become the transference object.

Eventually, Ethan spoke of growing up with a father who was intellectually rigorous but emotionally invasive. "He wanted to know everything. Every mood I had, every stray thought, he'd pounce on it. I learned early on that the best way to keep myself was to stay outside of myself." In the analytic situation, I had become a different kind of threat: not interpretive like his father, but inviting in a way that made him feel psychically porous. He needed the boundary of narrative to feel protected. My attempts to offer containment without coherence—to simply be with him without structuring meaning—left him exposed.

I shifted my stance. I began to reflect on the process more explicitly: "I wonder if the way I wait with you feels like pressure — like I'm trying to make something happen." He nodded, relieved. "Exactly. It's like you're not saying anything, but somehow I still feel like I'm disappointing you." In making the dialectic visible, I began to re-establish trust. Together, we crafted a new rhythm—one that did not idealize silence or interpretive distance, but allowed for a shared awareness of how each moment was being received.

In time, Ethan began to allow more ambiguity into the room. He would still narrate, but with small detours: a phrase would trail off, a metaphor would appear. And in those moments, we could meet without either of us having to know exactly what was happening. He did not become a different kind of patient. But he no longer needed coherence to defend against containment. He began, slowly, to tolerate being felt with—not explained, not soothed, but accompanied—even when nothing quite made sense.

Temporality and the Pacing of the Dialectic

The dialectic of coherence and containment is not only spatial or structural—it is profoundly **temporal**. Clinical work unfolds in time, and the question of *when* to speak, interpret, or remain silent is as critical as *what* is said or unsaid. Ferenczi's emphasis on elasticity—his insistence that the analyst be attuned to the moment-by-moment shifts in the patient's readiness to feel or symbolize—prefigures this temporal sensitivity. He understood that psychic meaning cannot be delivered; it must arrive when the psyche is ready to metabolize it.

Timing errors in analysis are often experienced not as technical missteps but as profound relational ruptures. An interpretation that is accurate in content but premature in timing may feel to the patient like a re-enactment of past violations: a parent who *knew too much too soon*, a caregiver who imposed structure before safety. Conversely, an interpretation that arrives too late—after the affective window has closed—may be experienced as abandonment, as if the analyst failed to notice or care when something vital was available to be known.

Bion's (1962) emphasis on waiting without memory or desire speaks directly to this. He describes the analyst as holding a position of suspended readiness—not detached, but receptive, able to notice when the analytic field is ripening toward meaning. Timing here is not chronological but affective: coherence must be invited, not enforced, and containment must be elastic enough to stretch across moments when nothing seems to happen but everything is being prepared.

Daniel Stern's (1985) work on "present moments" in infant–caregiver interaction reinforces this perspective. He observes that micro-events—lasting mere seconds—carry disproportionate developmental weight when the parent's response is attuned in tempo as well as tone. Similarly, in psychoanalysis, therapeutic impact is often not located in grand interpretations but in the analyst's **timely modulation of presence**: the sigh that mirrors a patient's grief, the pause that lets something unspoken breathe, the phrase offered not too early and not too late.

The temporality of trauma also haunts this dialectic. Traumatic memories resist linear sequence and often return in fragments, images, or bodily states that feel timeless. As Laplanche (1999) argued, the enigmatic signifier—the adult message beyond the child's comprehension—creates a temporal disjunction that reverberates across the life span. In the clinic, this requires that the analyst not only track meaning but tolerate **asynchrony**—moments when the patient's affective time does not match narrative time. To insist on coherence in those moments is to violate the psychic tempo that trauma has fractured. Instead, the analyst must join the patient where they are: in the nonlinear, the paused, and the delayed.

Ferenczi's technique of "mutual elasticity" was an early experiment in synchronizing analytic tempo to the patient's psychic state. His willingness to shorten sessions, alter timing, or delay interpretation was less about permissiveness than about respecting the patient's **sovereignty over time**—an ethic of not forcing the psyche to process faster than it can bear. Modern analysts may hesitate to adopt Ferenczi's formal elasticity, but the underlying principle remains vital: **time must be felt**. The analyst must learn to pace with the patient's rhythms, to feel when meaning is near but not yet ready to emerge, and to sense when containment has lasted long enough to make symbolic reach possible.

This is where the dialectic becomes dynamic: coherence and containment are not fixed poles but evolving positions within an ongoing clinical process. The analyst's instrument is not just interpretation or presence, but timing—the discipline of waiting, the courage to enter, and the humility to exit the moment before it becomes too filled. In this way, Ferenczi's unfinished vision continues: not a technique, but a tempo. Not a procedure, but a pacing of care.

Micro-Vignettes: Subtle Shifts in the Dialectic

While extended clinical vignettes can illuminate the arc of therapeutic transformation, it is often in the smallest moments—gestures, hesitations, timing—that the dialectic between coherence and containment becomes most visible. The following micro-vignettes illustrate how subtle shifts in the analyst's stance can open or foreclose possibilities for meaning, depending on how they negotiate the patient's unspoken needs for being held or understood.

Micro-Vignette 1: The Interpretation That Waited

A patient, mid-sentence, broke off and looked out the window. "Never mind," he said. "It doesn't matter." I almost spoke—I had a formulation ready, something linking his trailing thought to a pattern we'd been tracking. But I felt the residue of his withdrawal—the closing of a door that hadn't been slammed, only quietly shut.

Instead of interpreting, I said, "It looked like something came, and then left again." He nodded. We sat in silence for a minute. Then he said, "I was going to say something about my father, but it felt too predictable — like I already knew what you'd say." His eyes returned to mine. "I didn't want it to become that kind of moment."

He needed the interpretation—but not yet. What he needed first was to feel that he could choose *when* and *how* to symbolize. In waiting, I had not withheld; I had made room.

Micro-Vignette 2: Holding without Drifting

A woman grieving the loss of her sister wept quietly in session. I sat with her, saying nothing. After several minutes, she looked up. "It helps that you're not trying to fix it," she said. Then, a pause. "But it also helps that I know you know what this is."

She needed both containment and coherence—but only in tandem. If I had spoken too soon, the grief might have sealed over. If I had said nothing, she might have floated alone in the pain. What helped was not the silence alone, but the analyst's attuned presence within it.

Micro-Vignette 3: The Correction

"I hate how much I'm crying," a patient said. "It's not rational." I gently offered, "Maybe the crying is a kind of truth — even if it's not logical."

She sat back. "That's better than what I was expecting," she said. "I thought you were going to ask what it reminded me of."

We laughed. Sometimes, coherence needs containment in order to be heard. And sometimes, containment *is* coherence—just not the kind that interprets.

These brief moments exemplify how the analyst's responsiveness to the patient's *temporal and symbolic needs* can shift the meaning of an intervention. Silence may soothe or abandon. Interpretation may clarify or colonize. The same act may be perceived as holding or intrusion, depending on the patient's capacity to tolerate meaning, presence, and symbolization. Clinical artistry lies in sensing which moment requires what—and bearing the ethical risk of getting it wrong.

Coda: The Dialectic as Ethical Listening

To reread Ferenczi through the dialectic of coherence and containment is to reorient psychoanalytic work not around technical mastery, but around relational risk. It is to treat the analytic setting not merely as a space for interpretation or reverie, but as a **field of tension**, where the analyst must constantly re-balance the urge to make meaning with the necessity of preserving the patient's psychic tempo.

This is not a call to therapeutic neutrality nor to therapeutic disclosure. It is a call to therapeutic discipline—a way of being that remains attuned to when the patient's need is for coherence that makes the self intelligible and when it is for containment that preserves the self from disintegration. In Ferenczi's work, we find the early scaffolding of this ethic: not in his theoretical architecture alone, but in his procedural daring, his refusal to insulate himself from the countertransference, and his capacity to be affected without losing his clinical bearing.

The dialectic becomes particularly urgent in an era of therapeutic culture that prizes narrative resolution. In contemporary discourse, trauma is often framed as something to be named, spoken, and worked through—a kind of cathartic coherence that risks reproducing the very violence Ferenczi warned against. The pressure to "tell one's story" can mirror the adult seducer's pressure to *know* the child, to render the inchoate into legible form. Analysts today must remain alert to how even our most compassionate efforts can become forms of epistemic dominance.

But there is equal risk in the counter-movement: the retreat into open-ended listening as a moral posture, where the analyst idealizes non-intrusiveness and disavows the patient's hunger for shared understanding. The patient who pleads not to be left alone with their affect—not to drown in the analyst's reverent silence—reminds us that containment, if unaccompanied by symbolic resonance, can become its own form of negation.

In this light, the dialectic of coherence and containment becomes not simply a clinical rhythm, but an ethical and developmental imperative. It reorients the analyst's task from mastering technique to inhabiting tension—to listening in a way that protects the patient's timing, safeguards symbolic authorship, and responds without colonizing.

This reframing of Ferenczi's legacy offers at least three implications for contemporary practice. First, it highlights the danger of premature interpretation not only in trauma work, but in ordinary moments of therapeutic urgency, where the analyst may be pulled to name what must first be held. Second, it clarifies the analytic stance needed in dissociative or fragmented states: one of disciplined containment that does not retreat from meaning, but waits until meaning can be co-constructed without coercion. And third, it suggests that therapeutic action often lies not in what is said, but in the analyst's capacity to remain attuned to the patient's psychic tempo—to sense when coherence might heal and when it might harm. These dynamics also have implications for training and supervision, where the pressure to "know" the patient's meaning may overshadow the need to help the supervisee tolerate uncertainty and sustain relational presence over interpretive accuracy. Kuchuck (2021) underscores how the analyst's ability to tolerate ambiguity and resist premature knowing is often what supervisees struggle with most—particularly when affective intensity threatens to exceed symbolic reach.

Ferenczi's final reflections—on tact, elasticity, and analytic tenderness—remain unfinished not only because his life ended abruptly, but because they ask something ongoing of us. To stay in the trembling space between knowing and not knowing. To resist the fantasy of clinical certainty. To recognize when the patient's silence, fragmentation, or delay is not a barrier to treatment, but an **ethical refusal**—a refusal to be prematurely known. And to offer coherence not as interpretation alone, but as a form of care that emerges only after containment has done its quiet, necessary work.

Ferenczi believed that the analyst must be emotionally affected by the patient's suffering—not as a loss of neutrality, but as an ethical stance rooted in mutual recognition and care.

7 The Wise Baby and the Unborn Self

This chapter explores the paradox of the "wise baby" as a clinical and symbolic figure: the prematurely knowing child who survives psychic overwhelm not through expression, but through dissociative stillness. Drawing on Ferenczi's *Confusion of Tongues* and integrating Winnicott, Bion, Eigen, Laplanche, Heidegger, and affective neuroscience, the chapter examines how early psychic life is shaped not only by trauma, but by the foreclosure of relational becoming. The "unborn self" is conceptualized as a state of suspended potential—a dissociated repository of disavowed affect, muted eroticism, and unformulated vitality. Clinical and philosophical reflections trace how this condition lives on in the analytic field as silence, somatic trace, or unworded pressure. Rather than viewing the wise baby as a developmental achievement or tragedy, the chapter treats it as an enduring internal figure that shapes both symptom and imagination. In this context, certain forms of psychic withdrawal may be understood as an **ethical refusal**—a resistance to symbolic capture when the surrounding field has not earned the right to receive the self. Analysis becomes not a restoration of lost self, but a witnessing of what was never allowed to form.

Myth as Prelude: Children Who Shouldn't Know

In the quiet echo of myth, we find anticipatory shadows of psychic structures yet to be named. Myths do not explain—they stage. They dramatize the impossibility of what the psyche must nevertheless endure. Before there was Ferenczi's wise baby, there was Athena, born fully formed from the head of her father; there was Chiron, the wounded healer, immortal yet unhealed; there was Horus, charged with the restoration of a shattered lineage before he could speak his own name. Each myth marks the psychic rupture of **a child prematurely burdened with the adult world**, a figure of knowing without the conditions to metabolize it.

Athena emerges not from the maternal body but from the paternal skull, armored and articulate. She is wisdom without infancy, cognition severed from nurture. She arrives not through developmental unfolding, but through rupture—a surgical delivery from thought itself. In psychoanalytic terms,

DOI: 10.4324/9781003715283-10

Athena is the fantasy of the prematurely mentalized child: articulate, sharp, contained, but missing the rhythms of emotional gestation. She knows too much and feels too little. She is what happens when the mind is born before the body has been held.

Chiron, too, is split by his own contradiction. An immortal centaur, gifted in healing arts, he is wounded by a poison he cannot cure. His knowledge comes not from education, but from pain. Chiron is wisdom etched into flesh, **the scholar whose curriculum was injury**. Like Ferenczi's wise baby, Chiron represents a paradox of psychic temporality: he knows more than anyone, but this knowledge is not post-developmental—it is the knowledge of survival, of learning in order not to perish. He becomes the teacher of gods and heroes but remains perpetually in agony. His wound is not symbolic; it is structural. He cannot unknow it, and it cannot heal.

And Horus—the divine child of Egyptian mythology—is tasked not only with avenging his father, Osiris, but with **reconstituting his dismembered body**. This is not justice; it is repair. Horus is the **restorative labor of a child born into chaos**, one whose selfhood must form in tandem with the project of holding together a traumatized world. His subjectivity is co-constructed with grief. In one version of the myth, Horus loses an eye in battle, only to have it magically restored—not as a return to wholeness, but as a permanent symbol of what was lost and made to function again. He is the emblem of psychic compensation: a child whose development is shaped not around play or discovery, but around the imperative to stabilize what preceded him.

These mythic children are not simply figures of early greatness. They are **structural dramatizations of the cost of knowing too soon**. In each, there is a breach in the symbolic order—a bypassing of becoming. They do not grow into their knowledge; they awaken inside it. Their stories reveal the psychic price of this precocity: isolation, pain, fragmentation, and deferred integration. They are not held into their roles; they are thrust into them. They survive not through regression, but through a kind of brilliant foreclosure.

In this way, myth functions not only as metaphor but as **proto-psychoanalysis**—mapping, long before clinical theory, the emotional topologies of paradoxical subjectivity. Athena's origin from the father's head is a symbolic foreclosure of maternity and the denial of vulnerability. Chiron's unhealable wound speaks to the impossibility of symbolic containment when pain becomes the site of knowledge. Horus' task of reassembly renders visible the burden placed on children who must act as emotional scaffolding for those who failed to hold them.

The psychoanalytic frame allows us to translate these mythic patterns into clinical and developmental terms—but we must first sit with the elemental clarity of the myths themselves. Each one offers a **psychic architecture of premature knowledge**—where subjectivity is not built from within, but **assigned from without**, leaving the interior inchoate. These children do not develop within containing structures; they *are the structure*. They become the language their culture lacked.

It is no accident that these myths are ancient. They represent, across cultures, a recurring anxiety about **the child who exceeds their station**—not through rebellion, but through forced accommodation. Their stories surface where cultural systems intuit that certain forms of knowing should not arrive without touch, without holding, without time. The myths mark not only an event, but a warning: that wisdom without infancy, healing without healing, and restoration without mourning create fractures in the soul that will later require a different kind of narrative, a different kind of witness.

It is precisely in the aftermath of these fractures that Ferenczi's wise baby enters the analytic canon—not as a symbol, but as a **structure**. The child who must bear what cannot be borne, who knows what they were not yet built to know. In what follows, we will track this structure as it unfolds clinically, theoretically, and symbolically. But let us begin with the myths not simply as poetic prelude, but as **reverberating residues**—the prehistory of the paradox.

The Wise Baby: Ferenczi's Inverted Subject

Ferenczi's *Confusion of Tongues* (1933) marks one of the most radical moments in the psychoanalytic tradition: the analyst turning away from a model of fantasy as defense and toward a theory of real trauma enacted within the very relational fabric meant to safeguard development. In that paper, Ferenczi describes how a child—confronted with adult seduction, violence, or overwhelming affect—abandons their own childish language and assumes the adult's symbolic code. They **speak the language of the adult** not because they understand it, but because they must. This is not empathy; it is a forced migration of the self into the other's unmetabolized world. Ferenczi names the child who responds with care and mentalization in the face of overwhelming adult need the *wise baby*—a formulation at once poetic and diagnostic.

The wise baby is **not precocious by nature, but by necessity**. They are not developmentally ahead, but relationally orphaned—compelled to survive not by retreat, but by taking up space they should never have been asked to occupy. They observe when they should be immersed, intuit when they should be clumsy, and contain when they should be exploding. Their capacity to appear empathic or knowing is not the fruit of nurturance, but a defensive adaptation to the absence of containment. What looks like maturity is often **a concealed form of dissociation**: an observing ego formed prematurely, not to reflect internal states, but to register and manage the unintegrated states of the adult other.

This is the first inversion: **the child as container of the adult's affect**. The architecture of development flips. Rather than the adult holding the child's emotional turbulence, the child begins to absorb the disavowed affect of the adult. They do not process it—there is no space to. They **house it**, unintegrated and unformulated, often with no narrative frame. Their self begins to organize around this task: not to be seen, but to see; not to be mirrored, but to mirror; not to ask, but to attune. Their inner world becomes an **archive of emotional debris** that belonged to someone else.

Here, **Foucault's genealogy of power and knowledge** becomes clinically poignant. The child does not enter into knowledge through play, through desire, through gradual assimilation. They are **installed into knowledge** as a function of power: the adult's unreflected trauma demands representation, and the child becomes the site of that representation. This is **discursive violence**, not developmental achievement. To know becomes to survive, and in surviving, the child enters a symbolic order that was never meant for them. They are subjectified not through recognition, but through appropriation.

This is also a profoundly **ethical failure**, which **Levinas's philosophy of the face** helps us articulate. Levinas proposes that subjectivity is born not in cognition, but in *being-for-the-other*—in the moment one becomes responsive to the vulnerability of another's face. The wise baby, however, is placed into this position *before* they themselves have been seen. Their ethical subjectivity is demanded before it is formed. They become a self **not through being witnessed**, but through having to witness. The structure of ethical becoming is reversed.

This second inversion—the demand to witness before being witnessed—establishes the core paradox of the wise baby. They are **psychically compelled to form an observing position** before they have any egoic infrastructure capable of integrating what is seen. This does not produce insight. It produces a split: the self becomes a location where unprocessed truths accumulate, dissociated from affect, from language, from play. The child knows—but they cannot feel what they know. This form of knowing is not developmental; it is **epistemological trauma**.

Importantly, this kind of premature knowledge is **not merely cognitive**. It includes sexual knowing, emotional knowing, relational knowing. The child knows too early what betrayal looks like, what seduction feels like, what rage sounds like. They may not be able to name it, but they begin to organize themselves around it. They enter what **Laplanche** would call the space of the *enigmatic signifier*—signs that come from the adult world, laden with sexual or affective intensity, but without translation. These signs **colonize the child's symbolic field**. They become languages the child must speak in secret, often through enactment, through fantasy, through bodily gesture.

We might say that the wise baby does not learn language; they are **occupied by it**. They become fluent in the unspeakable. This links closely to **Wittgenstein's insight** that the limits of our language are the limits of our world. When meaning is imposed rather than discovered, the subject does not find speech—they find **compliance**. And where speech cannot express the depth of affective intrusion, **silence becomes the only ethical position**. The wise baby is often profoundly mute in their core affective life—not because they do not feel, but because **their feeling has no relational permission to exist**.

This is the soil in which **the false self**, as Winnicott would later articulate it, begins to grow—not as a mask over the true self, but as a **structure of intersubjective survival**. The wise baby develops a self that does not misrepresent, but **represents what was required**, what was demanded, what was feared. Their apparent strength is often **a holding pattern**, a form of internalized adultification. They are not "mature for their age." They are *reversed in their architecture*. They grow from the outside in.

Clinically, these patients often present with exquisite perceptual sensitivity, intellectual fluency, and a tendency to dissociate under relational pressure. Their early symptom is often **emotional clairvoyance**—they can detect others' needs and states with uncanny precision, but are largely disconnected from their own. Their stories frequently center on early caregiving roles, absent caregivers, or traumatic attunement to adult distress. But more subtle forms exist too: the analyst may feel persistently **witnessed by the patient**, even as the patient remains elusive. The wise baby watches as a way of existing; they do not enter the room so much as **hover above it**, registering everything.

To engage such patients is not to interpret too soon, but to **uninstall the premature interpretive structure** they've built. It is to create a space where knowing is not required, where observation is not the price of safety. The analyst must bear the paradox that the patient cannot yet tolerate: **to feel without needing to fix, to exist without being useful**. This is a reversal of the reversal—a slow return to a subjectivity that is not performative, but relational.

In what follows, we will explore the consequences of this psychic architecture: how it shapes affective life, how it distorts temporality, how it constructs paradoxes in embodiment, witnessing, and symbolic enactment. But the core remains: the wise baby is not a poetic image—it is a **developmental structure of survival**. One that turns the child into a knower at the expense of their capacity to be known.

Ontological Fallout: Being without Becoming

If the wise baby is a subject who knows before they can feel, what then becomes of the emotional life suspended beneath that knowledge? What becomes of the self whose first act is not being, but containment? The consequence is not only psychic overdevelopment in one domain and underdevelopment in another—it is a more fundamental disturbance: a **crisis of becoming**. The child becomes structured not around presence, but around a substitution for presence. What results is not the absence of self, but a **self that was never allowed to unfold into being**. A self whose aliveness is organized around the need to manage aliveness itself.

This is not simply a dissociative response to trauma. It is a disturbance in the basic **architecture of subjectivity**, in which existence is not the outcome of relational holding, but the artifact of compensatory survival. This is what **Winnicott** means when he writes that "there is no such thing as a baby"—only a baby-and-caregiver, a dyadic unit in which the infant's subjectivity emerges in response to being held, mirrored, and protected. The wise baby subverts this structure. Their subjectivity does not emerge from being held, but from holding. Their selfhood forms in response to the absence of the other's capacity to contain. What should have been offered to them is instead

organized around them. They are a subject formed in the empty space where holding should have been.

This leads to what we might call an **ontological inversion**: the self becomes a structure of **negative containment**. Not a person with needs, but a location where others' needs were housed. Not a subject of experience, but a facilitator of others' experience. This inversion produces a paradox: the self is present, yet fundamentally uninhabited. A **container without content**, or worse—a container filled with unprocessed remnants of others' emotional debris.

This description resonates with **Bion's** theory of **unmentalized affect**, where early experiences—particularly traumatic or overwhelming ones—cannot be symbolized and thus remain in the psyche as **beta-elements**: raw, sensory-affective fragments that cannot be dreamt, digested, or thought. These fragments circulate without integration, leading to disorganized mental life, or what **Ogden** later calls "undreamt dreams"—states of experience that were never metabolized, never permitted to become part of a usable inner world. The wise baby is not a dreamer; they are a **witness to the dreams of others**, including dreams that the others disavowed. They accumulate experience that does not belong to them and yet defines them.

Michael Eigen offers a language of depth here, describing how trauma can leave behind not just wounds, but **zones of unbeing**. He writes of patients who are alive, but not living—who survive in a muted register of experience, suspended in a state of emotional half-life. This is not repression; it is a kind of **existential muteness**, in which the subject exists without fully inhabiting their own interior. Their affect is not defended against, but **never allowed to take shape** in the first place. What Eigen calls "the feel of being" is missing not because it was crushed, but because it was never received. The wise baby, in this sense, becomes the site of an **unborn emotional life**—a life displaced by knowledge, by observation, by adultified survival.

Yet this absence does not remain inert. It becomes a structure. **Kernberg's theory of affective integration** helps us see how. In his work on borderline personality organization, Kernberg describes how early trauma leads to **splitting** of affect: positive and negative emotions are stored in separate compartments of the psyche, unable to be synthesized into a coherent emotional narrative. More profoundly, Kernberg argues that **love and aggression** are not secondary developments—they are **supraordinate constituents**, from which the drives and ego itself derive. This means that early disruptions in the integration of these affects are not simply emotional difficulties—they are **developmental injuries at the level of psychic formation**.

In the case of the wise baby, the affects are not only split; they are **disowned entirely**. Because the affective life was not permitted symbolic expression, it becomes suspended, often absorbed into the needs and emotions of the adults around them. Kernberg's love-aggression axis is not merely dissociated—it is externally invested. Love becomes care for others; aggression becomes internalized self-criticism, shame, or despair. What remains is a **psychic cavity**—a **void** where integration should have occurred.

We might call this void a **negative emotional core**—not a blank space, but a receptacle for unintegrated, unspoken, and unclaimed feelings. This inner blackness is not neutral. It **absorbs** affect the way a black hole absorbs light—without reflection, without return. And this void does not remain sealed; it subtly organizes behavior, sensation, fantasy, and relational style. The subject may not speak of emptiness, but they **act it out**, often through withdrawal, perfectionism, or compulsive caretaking.

Here, **Heidegger's concept of thrownness (*Geworfenheit*)** becomes clinically useful. The wise baby is **thrown** into a world they are not developmentally prepared to make meaning from, and they respond not with curiosity but with duty. Heidegger's notion of *Befindlichkeit*, or "state-of-finding-oneself," points to the affective mood through which one encounters the world. For the wise baby, this mood is not joy, exploration, or even fear—it is **attunement without anchoring**, a being-for-others that precedes being-for-self. Their "finding" of themselves happens within the emotional topography of another's psyche. They begin **not in their own affect**, but in the field of another's disorganization.

Merleau-Ponty takes this further in his phenomenology of embodiment. For him, the body is not a thing one has, but **a location through which the world is lived**. But the wise baby's body is never primarily their own. It is read by others before it is experienced from within. It is touched too early, burdened too soon, or needed in ways that collapse the self-world distinction. Their body becomes a **site of relational instrumentation**, rather than a subjective presence. As adults, such individuals often experience profound alienation from their own bodily states—alternating between hypersensitivity and numbing, between compulsive attunement and absence.

The long-term consequence is a **topology of paradox**: a subject whose survival required them to both be and not be. They are present enough to observe, to perform, to anticipate—yet absent from their own affective depth. They are emotionally fluent on behalf of others, but mute in their own interior. They are sensitive to nuance, yet incapable of tolerating the ambiguity of feeling. This is not a personality disorder. It is a **developmental structure built atop foreclosure**—a life lived adjacent to itself.

Clinically, these patients often struggle with deep feelings of fraudulence. Not because they are false, but because **they have never experienced themselves as real in the context of being seen**. The analyst's task here is not to reflect, interpret, or even soothe. It is to hold open the space of **non-demanding presence**—to become, perhaps for the first time, the one who does not need them to know, to fix, to contain. The therapeutic stance becomes not a mirror, but a **womb-like field**—a relational surround within which **being can re-emerge slowly, tentatively, paradoxically**.

In this chapter's unfolding, we have begun with myth, moved into Ferenczi's structural clinical insight, and now traced the ontological consequences of premature knowledge. But what of the specific psychic functions that take shape to manage this paradox? What of the ego that observes too soon, and in doing so, fractures the capacity to feel? To that, we now turn.

The Prematurely Formed Observing Ego

In classical developmental theory, the observing ego is the fruit of maturation. It enables reflection, modulation, and mentalization; it is the psychic space from which the self becomes available to itself. But in the architecture of the wise baby, this function arrives too soon. It emerges not as an achievement of integration, but as a defense against unintegrated experience. The observing ego is **prematurely erected**, not to facilitate thought, but to survive it.

This early emergence of an observing function reflects Ferenczi's understanding of traumatic adaptation: the child, in the face of overwhelming affect, displaces their experiencing self with an **internal witness**. They cease being the one who feels and become the one who notices. This noticing is not curious—it is protective. It detaches rather than reflects. It is not introspection; it is evacuation. In this premature configuration, the observing ego becomes not a psychic stabilizer, but a **barrier to immersion**—a shield that ensures survival by never quite letting the self arrive.

In some clinical contexts, this structure appears as early philosophical abstraction, uncanny verbal precision, or compulsive self-monitoring. In others, it emerges as mystical derealization: the patient who is present, but always beside themselves. One patient, during a ketamine-assisted session, entered what he described as a state of cosmic union. "I am God," he said, suffused with a sense of timeless interconnectedness. But the moment he thought the sentence—*I am God*—he described something cleaving. "As soon as I had the thought," he said, "I knew I was no longer it. I was watching myself being it. And it was over."

This vignette encapsulates the tragedy of the wise baby's observing ego: **to observe is to separate**. The very act of naming collapses the state of being. In healthy development, the capacity to symbolize expands the range of experience. But when this capacity precedes containment, it becomes a site of collapse. The self is no longer a wave of feeling—it becomes a particle of thought.

This parallels the **observer effect in quantum mechanics**, particularly in the double-slit experiment. When unobserved, a photon behaves like a wave, moving through multiple possibilities simultaneously. But once measured—once observed—it collapses into a particle, with fixed position and velocity. The act of observation changes the phenomenon itself. The child who forms an observing ego too early becomes like that photon: a being of diffuse potential who collapses into rigidity under the gaze—especially the gaze internalized as necessary for survival.

In the case of the wise baby, this observing gaze is not benign. It is constructed in response to being watched too closely, too intrusively, or not at all. The child watches themselves because **no one else can be trusted to do so**, or because the act of being seen has itself become unbearable. In this dynamic, the self is never simply lived—it is always **monitored**. Experience becomes an event *to be managed*, not inhabited.

Karen Barad's concept of intra-action expands this insight. In her theory of agential realism, the observer is not separate from what is observed. Rather, the act of observing constitutes the phenomenon itself. Applied clinically, this means that premature observation is not merely reflective—it is formative. The wise baby's ego is shaped not from developmental unfolding, but from the **need to produce legibility under conditions of incoherence**. They observe themselves in order to appear, to be known, to organize the chaos around them. The observing ego is not a tool; it is a **survival scaffold**.

This structure creates a persistent clinical paradox. Patients with prematurely developed observing egos often struggle in treatment, not because they lack insight, but because **they observe instead of feel**. They monitor the transference, track the analyst's phrasing, and analyze their own dreams before the analyst can respond. They are exquisitely attuned, yet psychically unmoored. They hover just outside their own affective life. The analyst often feels *seen but not reached*, involved in a process that is happening *around* rather than *with* the patient.

In these cases, the therapeutic task is not to dismantle the observing ego, but to **displace its centrality**. The analyst must become a second observer—not one who intrudes, but one who *delays the need for observation*. In this relational space, the patient can begin to feel without having to immediately watch themselves feel. Observation becomes co-constructed rather than prematurely imposed. This is what makes the analyst a **quantum partner**, not a mirror: one whose gaze alters the system by holding rather than collapsing it.

The clinical posture here must be exquisitely attuned, but **non-demanding**. Interpretation, if offered too soon, becomes another gaze that collapses experience into commentary. What the patient needs is not to be interpreted, but to be *allowed to exist unobserved long enough to experience themselves*. In this sense, the analyst enacts a **corrective delay**—a holding in time that enables what was previously unformed to be formed, not watched.

Over time, the observing ego can shift from a defensive scaffold into a reflective capacity. The patient learns to inhabit feelings without dissociating into commentary. They begin to weep without naming the tears, to rage without explaining the rage, to feel joy without the caveat of irony. These are not breakthroughs; they are **slow re-entries** into affective presence. The self begins to trust its own immersion.

To say it differently: the patient becomes **both wave and particle**. Observed and immersive. Known and lived. The paradox of the wise baby does not resolve—it **opens**. What was once a survival distortion becomes a psychic capacity: to know oneself without annihilating the experience of being.

This is the long arc of analytic repair—not to dissolve the observing ego, but to **rebirth the self beneath it**. To permit a being to arrive *after* the time in which they were made to perform. And to witness, slowly, as that being begins to observe not from fear, but from presence.

Echoes across Disciplines: Paradox and Premature Knowledge

The structure of the wise baby—the prematurely burdened subject, the knower without containment, the being cleaved by observation—does not belong to psychoanalysis alone. It recurs, like a strange loop, across disciplines: in logic, mathematics, quantum mechanics, linguistics, and aesthetics. Each offers a formal language for the psychic paradox we've been exploring. Together, they suggest that the wise baby is not only a developmental trauma structure, but a topological reality—a recursive system caught between immersion and self-reference, experience and observation, presence and disappearance.

This section draws five such parallels, each accompanied by a clinical vignette. The goal is not to flatten the psychoanalytic into the metaphorical, but to show that these structural logics are isomorphic: different disciplines naming the same rupture in different tongues.

Russell's Paradox: The Set That Contains Itself

In formal logic, Russell's Paradox destabilized naïve set theory by asking: Does the set of all sets that do not contain themselves contain itself? If it does, it shouldn't; and if it doesn't, it should. This self-referential contradiction is not just a logical error—it is a collapse of structural coherence when a system is asked to hold what it cannot metabolize.

So too with the wise baby, whose subjectivity is asked to hold the adult's unprocessed affect. They become self-designed to house what should have contained them. The contradiction is not cognitive—it is ontological.

Vignette: A child spends every therapy session making lists of his mother's emotions: "Monday she was sad, Tuesday she was angry…" When the analyst asks, "And how did you feel?" the child looks confused. "I wasn't really there," he says. "I was making sure she was okay." He is the set that contains the set that was meant to contain him.

Douglas Hofstadter's *strange loop* concept helps us here. The child becomes an entity defined by recursive self-containment—a loop of survival built around paradox. "I exist only because I held what undid me." The strange loop is a form that points to itself, turning the psychic architecture of the wise baby into a Möbius strip of relational inversion.

Klein Bottle: The Inside That Is Outside

A Klein bottle is a topological object that has no inside or outside. Its surface loops into itself such that interior and exterior are continuous, indistinguishable. Unlike the Möbius strip, which exists in three dimensions, the Klein bottle can only be fully realized in four-dimensional space. In ordinary space, it appears self-intersecting—because the topology it expresses defies the dimensionality of its environment.

This is the psychic shape of the wise baby: a subject whose boundaries were never made legible. In developmental terms, they were never allowed to be inside—to be held. Their containment was permeable, often reversed. They become porous, overexposed, and unlocatable.

Vignette: A woman describes feeling "too hollow but also too full." She speaks of relationships as "spilling into me," but when alone, she feels like "an empty room with the lights on." Her dreams often feature houses with no doors, just mirrors. In session, she flips between fusion and cold detachment. There is no middle. She lives without psychic skin.

Agamben's theory of the *zone of indistinction* helps us here. The wise baby is a sacred-excluded figure, occupying a threshold between roles—child/adult, seen/hidden, subject/object—but claimed by none. Their inner world is an echo chamber of relational reversal. Like the Klein bottle, their form cannot be housed in the symbolic dimensions available to them.

Jakobson's Shifter: I/You Without Anchor

In linguistics, a shifter is a word like "I," "you," or "here," whose meaning depends entirely on context. It cannot be understood in isolation; it is relationally anchored. Without another speaker, the shifter dissolves.

The wise baby becomes a shifter without anchoring. They adopt adult positions—caretaker, empath, observer—but without the relational context that gives those roles meaning. Their "I" is often an echo, not a voice.

Vignette: A man recounts a memory of being scolded in school: "You're just sitting there, and suddenly the teacher screams your name." He pauses. "I mean, I guess I mean me." His narrative shifts uncontrollably between first and second person. In session, he speaks as if overheard, haunted by an absent listener. He floats in pronouns, unable to land.

Wittgenstein reminds us that the meaning of language is use—but the wise baby's use is mimicry, not ownership. Their words do not express; they substitute. Language becomes a survival syntax, devoid of shared subjectivity.

Musical Dissonance Without Resolution

In tonal music, dissonance creates emotional tension. It signals movement and invites expectation. But it requires resolution to feel complete. Without resolution, dissonance becomes unnerving—an ache with no arc.

The wise baby's affective life is a perpetual suspended chord. Their sadness does not weep; their rage does not ignite. They live in emotional prelude—forever winding up without release.

Vignette: A young woman describes her panic attacks: "It starts like a buzz in my chest, like I'm waiting for something bad to happen, but it never does." In session, her affect crescendos but never reaches its peak. Her pain hums, unresolved. She leaves therapy saying, "It's like something should have happened... but didn't."

Kristeva's theory of abjection reframes this tension. The wise baby's affect is not repressed—it is unbearable. It must be expelled to survive, but never metabolized. Their emotional chords hum in the air, unresolved because they were never permitted to play.

Schrödinger's Cat: Observation as Collapse

In quantum mechanics, Schrödinger's cat is both alive and dead until observed. The act of observation collapses the quantum state into one possibility. Until then, the system exists in superposition—a state of potential multiplicity.

The wise baby lives with this paradox psychologically. When alone, they are vibrant, immersed, wave-like. But when seen—especially when observed as children—they collapse into roles, into survival configurations. Observation kills spontaneity.

Vignette: A man describes sex as "the only time I feel real," but also says, "I have to be alone after, because if someone sees me too closely, I disappear." He recounts a fantasy of being watched—but only through a one-way mirror. "If they see me and I see them seeing me," he says, "it's over. I go blank." The analyst becomes a quantum observer; the session, a wave function waiting to collapse.

Karen Barad's theory of *intra-action* extends this: observer and observed are not separate entities—they co-constitute reality. The analyst's gaze does not reflect the patient; it creates possibilities of being. The wise baby, prematurely observed, was never permitted to form in superposition. They became a particle before they could be a wave.

Refracting the Paradox

Each of these metaphors points to the same core structure: a self that cannot tolerate the terms of its own emergence. The wise baby is not an error of development, but a recursive knot—an entity whose presence destabilizes the categories through which presence is defined. They are:

- A set that contains what they should contain
- A boundary without inside or out
- A speaker without anchoring
- A chord without resolution
- A wave collapsed into a particle too soon

These are not metaphors of deficit. They are metaphors of topological paradox—twisted spaces where logic bends around the conditions of psychic survival. They show us that the wise baby's difficulty is not only in their past, but in the form of their subjectivity itself.

Psychoanalytic work with such patients is thus not an act of translation, but of spatial repair. The analyst does not explain the paradox—they enter it. They hold it open. They inhabit the Klein bottle without trying to invert it. They delay the collapse of the wave. They tolerate the suspended chord.

Only then can the wise baby begin to feel what they know, speak from within what they once observed from without, and tolerate a self that is neither resolved nor erased—but lived.

Secret Theaters: The Return of Dissociated Affect

The paradox of the wise baby is not resolved by time. What was disavowed in development does not vanish—it returns, not as integrated memory, but as symbolic residue, often in the form of solitary or secret enactments. These are not symptoms in the medical sense; they are theaters—staged spaces where dissociated affect is given form, often without conscious understanding. Sexuality, addiction, and fantasy do not merely express desire or defense; they are containers for unintegrated psychic fragments—emotional particles that could not find a relational home, now made to orbit privately.

These theaters are born of absence. The wise baby, having become the holder of others, displaces their own affective life into symbolic domains where no witnessing is required. Their emotional life returns in disguised form: not toward another, but within carefully managed rituals of self-stimulation, solitary fantasy, or controlled transgression. This is the third inversion: what should have been held by the other is now held in private—not as integration, but as recursive expression.

Sexuality as Private Regression

Sexuality often becomes the most vivid stage upon which these fragments of the self return. Not because it is inherently traumatic, but because it offers a field of dissociation and surrender—a symbolic space where the child's original paradox—knowing without being—can be replayed. Many wise-baby patients experience sex not as mutuality, but as a scene in which they can undo their observing ego and regress into affective states otherwise inaccessible.

One patient described his sexuality as a "ritual space," where he could be "helpless, held, or punished." In the analytic setting, he was articulate, hyperattuned, and resistant to affect. But in sexual fantasy, he became soft, wordless, feelingful. "It's the only place I don't have to be useful," he said.

This is not pathology. It is a kind of ritualized re-mothering—a private attempt to symbolically re-enter states of dependence, affectivity, and even preverbal aliveness. Bollas's concept of the *unthought known* is especially salient here. These are not memories but felt truths that precede articulation—states the psyche continues to organize around, despite never having been symbolically metabolized.

Addiction as Solitary Soothing

Where sexuality often facilitates symbolic regression, addiction may serve as a pseudo-container. Repetitive rituals—drinking, drug use, compulsive scrolling, eating, exercising—become self-witnessing loops, replacing what should have been external regulation with internal, numbed rhythm.

A woman described her drinking as "a way to fold time in on itself." She drank alone, never to excess. "It's like making a soundproof box around myself. It keeps everything else out, but also keeps me from leaking." When asked what would happen without it, she said: "Then I'd have to feel everything."

These behaviors are not driven by pleasure but by affective surplus without containment. They are defensive acts of internal sealing—places where feeling can be bracketed from relational exposure. Laplanche's theory of the *enigmatic signifier* offers a framework: early experiences saturated with adult affect—especially sexual or unregulated emotion—enter the child's psyche without translation and are later re-enacted not to remember, but to hold. Addiction is not the return of the repressed—it is the unprocessed made temporarily bearable.

Fantasy as Symbolic Re-entry

Fantasy becomes its own affective ecology—particularly in wise-baby structures, where the real relationship is saturated with performative demand. In fantasy, the patient is not observed. There is no gaze to collapse into. The fantasy becomes a space where dissociated affect can be projected, metabolized, and even witnessed—but only by the self.

One man described elaborate scenes in which he was abandoned, found, nursed, or punished. "I imagine it all in third person," he said. "I watch it happen like a film. It's not me, but it is." The fantasy returned him to states of injured dependency that never had a place in an actual relationship. He did not enter the fantasy to escape the real, but to symbolically re-enter what the real foreclosed.

These fantasies are not acts of avoidance. They are affective rituals—like dreams without dreamwork—through which the psyche attempts symbolic entry into previously unlivable states. The wise baby often cannot afford to feel in the presence of another. But in fantasy, affect becomes decoupled from relational collapse—and thereby becomes survivable.

The Private as Substitute for the Witnessed

Across sexuality, addiction, and fantasy, the same structural pattern recurs: affect that could not be felt in the relationship is displaced into solitary symbolic domains. These are not merely intrapsychic compromises. They are substitutes for what was never held. In each, we see the failure of what Jessica Benjamin calls *mutual recognition*. The self was never met in its subjectivity and thus retreats to sites where recognition is staged but never risked.

Benjamin's notion of *witnessing failure* is essential here. The wise baby's trauma is not merely the presence of overwhelming experience—it is the absence of a witness to that experience. As a result, they become both performer and audience, speaker and hearer. Their affective life is closed-circuit—looped through private theaters where safety and isolation become indistinguishable.

The Analyst and the Deferred Witness

Analytically, these secret domains should not be treated as mere defenses. They are symbolic survival zones—emotional sanctuaries constructed in the absence of witnessing. The analyst must not dismantle them, but approach them symbolically, with reverence. The task is not exposure, but accompaniment.

This analytic stance echoes Winnicott's concept of *transitional space*—a third area between inner and outer reality where the patient can experiment with presence. But it also requires what Eigen calls *reverberative containment*: the willingness to hold affective states without immediate interpretive capture. Not to make meaning of the scene too quickly, but to remain with the rhythm of feeling that had previously been exiled from the relationship.

These rituals—whether sexual, addictive, or fantasized—are not pathological regressions. They are developmental enactments, attempts to symbolically enter what was bypassed. In this sense, they are rituals of return. Not to trauma, but to the missing witness—the relational possibility that never materialized.

In the next section, we turn toward the archetype of rebirth—not as a metaphor for renewal, but as a psychic and relational event: the slow emergence of a self that was once used, now invited to appear. Not to be interpreted, but to be held.

From Initiation to Rebirth: Analyst as Second Witness

The wise baby is a psychic structure defined by premature knowing, affective foreclosure, and a relational absence so total that it installs the child into symbolic life before they are biologically or emotionally prepared. But if this condition is not resolved through insight, interpretation, or even memory, then what becomes of it? What is the clinical and existential path forward for a subject formed in reverse?

This section offers no solution. Rather, it turns to one of the oldest human motifs: **rebirth**. Not as a metaphor for regression or repair, but as a **structure of symbolic re-entry**—a second beginning for a self who was only half-born. To frame this process, we draw on religious ritual, shamanic initiation, and post-structural theory—not to romanticize rebirth, but to dignify its *psychic reality* in analytic work. For many patients, especially those organized around wise-baby structures, rebirth is not a return to innocence. It is a **first passage into inhabitable experience**, made possible only through the co-presence of an other who does not collapse or demand.

Shaman without Initiation

In many Indigenous cultures, the **wounded healer** is initiated through rupture—illness, vision, and near-death. Their trauma becomes a source of power, but only through **communal ritual** that translates pain into symbolic authority. The shaman is not a child performing for the adult's unmet needs; they are a **mediator of realms**, authorized and held by their community.

The wise baby resembles the shaman in their wound—but **lacks the initiation**. Their premature knowledge is not ritually metabolized; it is **privatized, disavowed, and unmet**. They carry the raw data of affective collapse without symbolic scaffolding. Where the shaman is welcomed into a new symbolic order, the wise baby is **left to perform symbolic labor for others without recognition**. They are shamanic without myth, gifted without permission, seen without being held.

What they need, in treatment, is not interpretation but **initiation by way of containment**: not into power, but into feeling, not into transcendence, but into presence.

Religious Structures of Rebirth

Religious traditions across cultures hold **rituals of rebirth** that echo this need for symbolic re-entry:

- In **Christianity**, baptism signifies a dying into water and a rising into new life. Christ, the child-God, is himself a figure of paradox: infinite and infantile, all-knowing and vulnerable. His crucifixion and resurrection embody a **ritual of annihilation and return**, with communal witnessing as the medium of transformation.
- In **Buddhism**, rebirth is not a return to the same life but a **karmic unfolding**. The subject is reborn not as a repetition but as a transformation—part of a chain of becoming in which suffering is not denied but refined.
- In **Hinduism**, the soul (ātman) undergoes multiple incarnations, each shaped by unresolved residues of affect, desire, and action. Rebirth is not an ideal—it is a **necessity born of incompletion** until integration occurs.

These narratives offer not solutions but **maps of paradox**. They mark the deep human intuition that some forms of knowing arrive **before the subject is ready** and that symbolic life must be revisited—not erased, but re-entered.

Foucault: Re-inscription, Not Return

If religious structures imagine rebirth through sacred rupture, **Foucault** offers a secular but equally potent lens. For Foucault, subjectivity is not a recovery of origins—it is a **re-inscription**. We do not return to what was lost; we **write ourselves into new symbolic orders**, often under conditions not of our choosing. Rebirth, then, is not regression—it is a **reconfiguration of the self within the field of power, gaze, and meaning**.

The wise baby, formed by unchosen inscription, needs not to go backward but to be **re-inscribed through witnessing**. The analyst does not restore a lost wholeness. They create the conditions under which **symbolic life can be reauthored**, this time with containment.

Barad: Co-Constitution and Intra-Action

Karen Barad's theory of agential realism extends this even further. Drawing from quantum physics, she argues that observer and observed are not separate. They emerge **through intra-action**—mutual constitution within a field. The subject is not fixed, but **brought forth through relational entanglement**.

This insight is central to analytic rebirth. The analyst does not reflect the patient's self; they **co-create the conditions under which that self may emerge differently**. The wise baby, whose original subjectivity was formed in isolation or misattunement, must now experience **a subjectivity formed with—not for—the other**.

The analyst becomes not an interpreter, but a **quantum partner**. Their gaze no longer collapses the wave-function of feeling. Instead, it allows **multiple states of being to remain in superposition** until the patient chooses, slowly, to inhabit one.

Rebirth as Temporal and Affective Re-Entry

In clinical terms, rebirth is not a moment. It is a **series of micro-entries into affective time**:

- The first time the patient cries in front of the analyst, and is not met with interpretation.
- The moment they regress into helplessness and are not used.
- The silence in which they are permitted to exist without commentary.
- The fantasy they share that is not decoded, but held.

Each is a small re-entry into a **chronology that was once foreclosed**. The analyst's job is not to direct this process, but to **hold open the gates of time**. To make possible what should have been possible then—*now*.

This holding is paradoxical: the analyst **must witness without collapsing**. They must not force integration, but rather allow **symbolic metabolization to occur over time**. This is **Loewald's temporal depth** in action: the capacity to hold the past not as memory, but as a field of affect **that may yet be reorganized in the presence of another**.

The Analyst as Ritual Function

Thus, the analyst becomes not a rescuer, but a **ritual function**: a **second witness** who appears not at the scene of the original trauma, but at the site where that trauma might finally be **symbolically transfigured**. They do not supply a narrative—they allow one to unfold. They do not re-parent—they **co-create a space where the patient can arrive, at last, without being used**.

The key gesture is **restraint**. The analyst must resist the urge to understand too quickly, to name too completely, to interpret too soon. Instead, they become a kind of **midwife of paradox**, holding the patient through **states of incoherence** that once had to be bypassed for survival.

In this role, the analyst restores not what was lost, but what was **never permitted to unfold**. The wise baby becomes a self—not through discovery, but through **inhabitation**. Their knowledge remains, but now it is accompanied by affect. Their language remains, but now it is tethered to embodiment. Their structure remains paradoxical—but now it is **witnessed, not hidden**.

To be reborn in this way is not to erase the past. It is to **symbolize what was lived without symbol**, to **feel what was known in absence**, and to **arrive in time after time has already begun**. This is not therapeutic insight—it is existential arrival. And it can happen only when someone else is there, not to demand, but to stay.

Conclusion: Paradox as Developmental Ethics

The figure of the wise baby does not resolve; it reverberates. Across this chapter, we have tracked its structure—from mythic antecedents to clinical enactments, from logical collapse to ritual rebirth. What began as a child prematurely forced to know without being has unfolded into a fully adult self whose psychic life remains shaped by this paradox: **presence born of absence, observation born of foreclosure, survival born of disowning aliveness**.

What psychoanalysis teaches us—if we are willing to follow it past the desire for integration—is that some structures are not meant to be resolved. They are meant to be **held open**. The wise baby is one such structure. It does not simply seek a return to what was lost, because what was lost never existed. What it seeks is something more complex: a space in which the **conditions of becoming** can be **co-constructed retroactively**—where containment, feeling, and witnessing can arrive *out of sequence*, not to correct history, but to allow its paradoxes to be lived.

This requires a shift in therapeutic posture. The analyst is not a healer restoring developmental continuity, nor a technician untangling knots. They are a **co-presence**, willing to **stand within contradiction** without trying to collapse it into meaning. They become, as **Levinas** might say, *the face that stays*—a witness who does not instrumentalize suffering, but holds it in ethical tension.

The ethics here are not moral. It is **temporal and existential**. It arises from the analyst's willingness to *not know*, to defer interpretation, to allow affect to emerge without being captured by language. It is what **Loewald** called the re-animation of psychic life through relational presence, what **Eigen** named the "feel of being" that emerges only when we are allowed to feel without function.

This is the ethics of **paradoxical development**—development that proceeds not through mastery, but through re-entry. Not through insight, but through slow symbolization of that which never had form. The wise baby does not need their early experience translated; they need the experience of being accompanied through what was once unaccompanied.

In this light, we might re-interpret Wittgenstein's dictum—"Don't think, look." To look is not to reduce; it is to be with. To bear witness to what cannot be said, and to stay near it. To feel the rhythm of what Kristeva called abjection—those elements of self and experience that were expelled to preserve coherence—and to recognize them as *belonging*, not because they fit, but because they persist.

Likewise, we might turn again to Hofstadter's "strange loop." The wise baby is a loop, not a line—a subjectivity that folds in on itself, produced not by narrative coherence but by recursive relation. They are the container of what should have contained them, the observer of what they were meant to feel, the caretaker of the affect that undid them. These are not errors; they are architectures of becoming under impossible conditions.

The analyst, then, does not offer linear restoration. They offer a *dwelling place* for paradox. They become the Klein bottle into which the patient can slowly step, not to be corrected, but to be lived. They become the silent chord that allows the dissonance to be heard without resolution. They become the delayed observer, allowing the patient to remain wave-like just long enough to trust collapse when it comes.

This work is quiet. It is not filled with breakthroughs or revelations. It is filled with slow pulses of presence, moments in which the patient, often for the first time, inhabits their affect without needing to explain it. It is in these moments that the wise baby becomes less wise, more feelingful. Less performative, more real. The paradox remains—but it is no longer hidden.

In this chapter, we have not sought to fix the wise baby. We have tried to think them to the edge of language, to track their movement through theory, myth, and metaphor, and to offer psychoanalysis not as a cure, but as a form of reverent companionship. A method of staying close to what never had a place.

For in the end, perhaps the most ethical thing we can do is not to resolve the paradox, but to love it into form.

8 Time-Bound Selves

Curation, Collapse, and the Temporality of the False Self

This chapter reframes the false self not merely as a defensive mask but as a structure of temporal regulation. Drawing on Winnicott, Loewald, Muñoz, Orange, and others, it argues that the false self often functions as an organizer of psychic time—anticipating, suspending, or stylizing experience in order to prevent symbolic collapse. Through clinical vignettes, this chapter explores three primary temporal structures: futurity, stylized stasis, and curated coherence. It then considers how the analyst's own temporal rhythm—tone, pacing, and interruption—shapes the intersubjective field and supports the patient's capacity to metabolize experience. This chapter closes with a reflection on how the false self may evolve, not by being dismantled, but by being held long enough to symbolically re-enter lived time. This temporal ethics invites the analyst to witness not only what the patient feels, but when and how that timing protects the possibility of selfhood.

Introduction: The False Self and the Architecture of Time

The false self has often been treated as a mask—a structure of deception, a compliance apparatus, a performance that conceals something more "real" beneath it. But what if we approached it not as a mask, but as a clock? A way of regulating not only emotion and visibility, but temporality itself?

Winnicott's theory of the false self has always carried a temporal undercurrent. In his 1974 paper *Fear of Breakdown*, he makes the startling claim that what the patient fears "has already happened." The dread that saturates the clinical encounter—a breakdown imagined as impending—is not future-oriented at all. It is a memory that has never been symbolized. The psyche holds it in suspension, and the false self organizes around that suspension. It is not just a mask for others; it is a holding structure for time that could not be lived.

In this light, the false self becomes more than a compromise formation. It is a **temporal architecture**, constructed to hold unformulated experience, to manage symbolic delay, to navigate an unspeakable past and an unlivable future. It freezes, performs, anticipates, and repeats—not to deceive, but to survive. In this chapter, I argue that one of the false self's most important—and least understood—functions is its regulation of psychic time.

DOI: 10.4324/9781003715283-11

For some patients, the false self organizes around **futurity**—a self devoted to perfection, discipline, and anticipation. Its vitality is tethered to an imagined future where spontaneous life will finally be permitted to unfold. For others, the false self creates a **timeless stasis**, stylized and dissociative, organized to avoid the movement of affect. Still others curate a coherent present in order to **displace a haunted past**—holding family secrets, inherited trauma, or early abandonment in coded rhythms and rehearsed narrative.

These time-bound structures are not peripheral to subjectivity. They are **its scaffolding**. They determine what can be symbolized, when, and in whose presence. The false self is not merely defensive—it is **temporal containment**. It holds back collapse not only of affect but of sequence, of meaning, of becoming. It allows life to unfold at a pace that does not overwhelm the symbolic order.

In the analytic encounter, these dynamics are not abstract. They shape countertransference, enactments, and the analyst's own temporal pressure: the wish to move forward, to slow down, to stop looping. Patients who organize around futurity may evoke in the analyst a desire to wait for something more "authentic," while those in stylized stasis may provoke impatience or despair. The analyst's own temporal ethics become central. To work with the false self is to tolerate **not knowing when—or whether—anything will change.**

This chapter traces three clinical portraits in which time itself is at stake. The first, a compulsively future-oriented patient, uses perfectionism as a structure of survival, deferring spontaneity to a fantasy of later authenticity. The second, trapped in an aestheticized stasis, uses the false self to avoid the terror of affective movement. The third curates a surface of coherence to prevent inherited trauma from flooding the symbolic field. In each case, the false self regulates not just affect but temporality—the rhythm by which experience can be lived, known, and shared.

To make sense of these dynamics, I draw not only on Winnicott but also on **Bromberg**, **Eigen**, **Muñoz**, **Orange**, **Sedgwick**, and **Loewald**. Together, they help us understand the false self as a **temporal ethic**: a way of staging experience, delaying collapse, and waiting for a world that can hold the unformulated. Rather than pathologize these strategies, I treat them as symbolic acts—recursive performances that both protect and disclose.

The analytic task is not to expose the real self beneath the false one. It is to recognize how the false self is organizing time—for the sake of coherence, survivability, and symbolic possibility. It is to enter the patient's temporal structure with care: to wait where they wait, to pause where they pause, to sense the rhythm by which a self might begin to appear. Not quickly, and never all at once.

Curating the Future: The False Self as Anticipatory Structure

He arrived like many high-functioning patients do—careful, articulate, even warm, but subtly rehearsed. His narrative was tight, his affect polished. What he wanted from therapy was "to become more spontaneous," he said, "to feel less like I'm performing my life." But as we spoke, it became clear that performance was not a layer to be stripped away. It was the structure that held everything in place.

His week was measured in deliverables, and his emotions in achievements. When I asked how he felt, he would tell me what he had *accomplished*. Even his moments of rest were optimized—curated to support his long-term goals. "Everything I do is for a future version of me," he said once. "A self I haven't met yet, but who I hope will be proud."

That sentence held the core of his psychic architecture: a false self organized not around hiding, but around **anticipating**. His vitality was tethered to **futurity**—a projected self who would justify the sacrifices of the present. In this logic, joy was deferred, vulnerability was unsafe, and present-moment contact was always slightly out of reach. The self was a performance, not of who he was, but of who he might someday be.

In these early months, he was attentive and grateful, but something remained elusive. Sessions were vivid but frictionless. I found myself waiting for something: a moment of unpreparedness, a break in cadence, a feeling that had not already been metabolized into insight. He could reflect endlessly—but rarely seemed *in* the material. His disclosures were moving but unmoored. It was as if he were narrating the story of someone he hoped to become intimate with.

Over time, what emerged was not resistance but **temporal misattunement**. He did not block the work—he was simply never quite *here*. He lived in a kind of performative prefiguration, a future anterior tense: "I will have become." His psychic structure was built to **delay the breakdown** he feared—not through avoidance, but through relentless optimization. What might have collapsed was managed through preparation. The false self here was not a defense against emotion; it was a mechanism for **scheduling it**.

When I pressed gently on this—asking what it would mean to live without such planning—he grew restless. "You don't understand," he said. "If I stop aiming at the future, I'll lose myself." There was no anger, just a sudden urgency. He was right. The self he had built was organized not around authenticity, but **arrival**. He could not simply collapse it. He needed someone to accompany its architecture—not to unmask it, but to understand it as **hope, protection, and exile**.

José Muñoz's notion of *queer futurity* helped me make sense of what I was seeing. In *Cruising Utopia*, Muñoz argues that queerness is not simply an identity but a horizon—an ideality, something not yet here but felt as a potentiality. "Queerness is not yet here," he writes. "We are not yet queer." In this frame, performance is not concealment but a **gesture toward the possible**. The curated self, then, is not necessarily inauthentic. It is *aspirational*. It performs for a future that may allow authenticity to exist.

This reframing softened something in my countertransference. I had been subtly waiting for this patient to become more "real"—to collapse into something raw, present, or unguarded. But this was my fantasy of the real. His performance was not evasion. It was a matter of **structure**, **longing**, and **temporal survival**. His false self was *symbolic labor*—a structure built to sustain hope in the absence of livable immediacy.

Over time, our work shifted. Rather than try to puncture the curation, I began to treat it as meaningful in its own right—a temporal ritual that both displaced and preserved something unspeakable. The question became not "What are you hiding?" but "What are you waiting for?" And more: "What happens to the self if what you're waiting for never comes?"

That question didn't land immediately, but it stayed in the room. Weeks later, he said, "I think I've always believed I'll be loved later when I'm more complete. But I don't know if later ever comes." The statement was quiet, almost theoretical. But it marked the first time he spoke from a place of temporal uncertainty rather than preparation. It was not a breakthrough. It was a **slippage**—a symbolic leak in the structure.

From here, we began to touch the affect beneath the ambition. He was not grandiose. He was terrified. The future was not his fantasy; it was his container. If he collapsed into the present, what would hold him? Who would? The false self, in this case, was the **only structure keeping psychic time from unraveling**.

In such cases, the analytic stance must shift. We do not ask for emotional immediacy. We do not valorize spontaneity. Instead, we listen for the patient's **temporal logic**—how they hold themselves together across sequences of becoming. The curated self is not the enemy of the real. It is its **temporal envelope**. And if we listen carefully, we may hear the rhythms of a future self knocking from inside it—not yet formed, but already rehearsing its arrival.

What emerged in the months that followed was not a breakthrough, but a slow reorganization of presence. The patient's elaborate self-presentation—once so tightly wound around imagined future approval—began to soften. He did not become more spontaneous in the usual sense. But he began to **risk ambivalence**. His statements grew less final. His interpretations, less rehearsed. When describing conflict or self-doubt, he no longer reflexively translated them into lessons. There was more air in the room.

In one session, after describing a moment of social awkwardness, he caught himself narrating it too neatly. "See?" he smiled. "I've already turned it into something teachable." Then he paused. "But actually, I just felt stupid. And I still do." It was an uncharacteristically unprocessed remark. A moment that did not point to the future, but sat in the present. It landed in the room not with drama, but with *resonance*.

In **Winnicott's** language, this may be understood as the emergence of "going on being." Winnicott's concern was never simply with pathology, but with *conditions*. The true self, for him, was not a thing, but a **temporal rhythm**—the capacity to live without constant interruption, without the premature need to perform or justify being. The false self, in this patient's case, had been a structure that pre-empted spontaneity by **locking the self into the**

future tense. Therapy, then, became a holding space not only for affect, but for **timing**. It permitted a slowing down of the compulsion to narrate forward.

Hans Loewald offers a powerful metapsychological framework here. For Loewald, symbolization is a temporal act—the transformation of raw experience into something that can exist in time, be revisited, remembered, and shared. Internalization, in his model, is not simply the ingestion of others but the integration of rhythm, tone, and responsiveness. The analyst is not a mirror, but a *symbolic partner in timing*. To internalize an experience is to bring it into temporal form.

My patient's forward-driven perfectionism had created a powerful **pre-symbolic defense** against internal collapse. The future was not just where success lived—it was where experience was stored, waiting to be lived *safely*. There was no room for symbolization in the present because the self was not permitted to fully arrive. Through our work, what began to develop was not insight but a **repatterning of psychic time**. He began to tolerate being "in between"—between feeling and understanding, between self and ideal, between gesture and coherence.

This transformation required my own temporal reorganization. At first, I had unwittingly colluded with the forward pace of his curation—waiting for something more "real" to emerge. But over time, I learned to **wait differently**, not for revelation, but for rhythm. I let myself be moved by the patient's pacing, his temporal self-states. I stopped listening for rupture and began listening for symbolic hesitation. The therapy began to hum at a different frequency—less about content, more about *timing*.

Donna Orange's work on presence is essential here. For Orange, therapeutic presence is not just emotional availability, but a **witnessing of temporality**—the patient's rhythm, their pauses, and their need to loop, delay, or displace. She writes of the "ethics of attunement," in which the analyst tolerates the patient's form without rushing it. This is not passive. It is deeply active, but in a different mode. One does not chase spontaneity, but makes it **livable**.

In this patient's case, the therapeutic presence that mattered most was not insight or interpretation, but **temporal containment**. When he began to question his relentless striving—"What if the future never comes?"—I didn't rush to reframe or reassure him. I waited with him in the tension of that uncertainty. Not knowing became something he no longer had to flee. His false self, which had once curated the future with architectural elegance, began to permit shadows, unfinished corners, and silent rooms.

Harry Stack Sullivan's notion of the self as "the pattern of reflected appraisals" also feels relevant here. For Sullivan, the self is not a core essence but a **relational artifact**—the accumulation of how one has been received. This patient's future orientation was not innate. It was a response to years of being praised for potential rather than presence. Therapy, then, became a counter-environment: a place where he could be met not for what he was becoming, but for what he was *being*—especially in moments that felt incomplete, dull, or unresolved.

This work does not end with catharsis. The false self does not dissolve. It shifts. It relinquishes its monopoly on meaning. The patient may still perform, still curate, still aim. But those gestures become more *symbolic,* less urgent. There is room for variation. The future stops being a rescue fantasy and becomes something more human—uncertain, open, survivable.

The final months of our work were marked by fewer grand declarations and more small moments of inhabitation. He would describe his week with less emphasis on achievement, more attention to tone. "It was kind of nothing," he'd say. "But it was mine." These were quiet claims of selfhood—not declarations of the true self, but **inhabited intervals**. In Loewald's terms, symbolic life had begun to flow. He was not performing for the future. He was *living in time*.

Freezing the Present: False Self and Timeless Collapse

He was beautiful, quiet, and exquisitely dressed. Every week, he arrived precisely on time, sat precisely where he always sat, and arranged his hands just so. There was nothing artificial about his presence, but something was conspicuously *curated*. His words were graceful, careful, articulate—but flattened, as if they had passed through a filter. He could describe emotional scenes in flawless detail without ever seeming to feel them. Pain, joy, hunger, disappointment—they all came in perfectly shaped vignettes. I found myself moved by the content, but never quite able to find him inside it.

From early on, I noticed a distinct kind of temporal stasis. Nothing in the sessions built on what came before. We weren't circling anything; we were orbiting. He told stories from childhood and recent life and described dreams and relationship ruptures, but the sessions never quite accumulated. There was no sense of deepening. Everything hovered, suspended in a present tense that felt simultaneously aesthetic and anesthetic.

I began to wonder if what I was encountering was not so much repression, but something like **stylized dissociation**—not avoidance, but precision. This was not someone refusing to be present. It was someone whose false self had become a *form of temporal suspension*. Time had been flattened. Symbolization, in the Loewaldian sense, was largely absent—not because he lacked language, but because language itself had become the structure of containment.

In **Winnicott's** 1974 *Fear of Breakdown*, he argued that the feared breakdown is not an impending catastrophe; it is a trace of something that could not be experienced at the time it occurred. In this patient, I began to suspect that his stylized, ritualized, and presentational self was structured precisely to **avoid triggering the non-experienced past**. The false self was not masking a more real self. It was *regulating time*. It held back affect not because it was repressive, but because it was the only form of continuity available.

In our early sessions, he described his childhood in metaphors: "It was like being in a museum," he said. "Everything was arranged, beautiful, and quiet.

But I didn't know where I was in the exhibit." His mother, an art historian, had filled the house with images of beauty and order. "Even our dinners looked like still lifes," he said. "There wasn't chaos. There just wasn't... anything." There were no overt traumas, no dramatic lacks. But there was a pervasive absence of symbolic connection. His caregivers had provided structure without presence. Recognition without attunement. Form without holding.

It became clear that his false self was not defensive in the classical sense. It was **ritualized**, almost devotional. He had curated his affective world with the same care his mother had curated her galleries—not to deceive, but to survive without collapse. To show feeling might have required first *finding it*. But the conditions for such a finding had never been present. What remained was a stylized, frictionless self, suspended in a timeless aesthetic.

Philip Bromberg's model of dissociative self-states helps make sense of this structure. For Bromberg, dissociation is not simply the splitting of experience, but the fragmentation of self-states that cannot be bridged symbolically. My patient had not repressed his feeling life—he had *quarantined* it into a self-state that was inaccessible in the analytic space. The self that appeared in session was not a performance of insincerity. It was a state curated to maintain coherence in the absence of shared temporal experience.

As I attuned more deeply to the analytic field, I noticed that even my breathing changed around him. I spoke more slowly. I paused longer between sentences. At times, I felt gently anesthetized—not bored, but tranquilized. I would leave our sessions feeling like I had been underwater. Not drowning, but suspended. It took some time before I realized this was not a case of countertransference resistance. It was **his temporal structure pulling me in**.

I began to understand this as a mutual enactment of **affective freeze**. He had found in me a partner willing to hold the pace. And I had unconsciously adapted to the structure of his false self. I did not challenge or interpret it. I mirrored its rhythm, its quiet, its form. In doing so, I became part of the holding—not yet transformative, but *non-intrusive*. This was not yet symbolization, but it was presence.

Michael Eigen writes about these spaces as "psychic pockets"—frozen zones in the psyche where experience could not unfold in time. He speaks of the analyst's task not as melting the freeze, but as **inhabiting it** long enough for its interior rhythms to emerge. In this case, I began to hear subtle variations: a phrase that sounded less polished, a gesture left unfinished, a sigh that felt unscripted. These were not ruptures. They were *micro-movements*. They suggested that the frozen self-state was not without life—it was simply operating at a tempo that resisted ordinary witnessing.

The turning point came not in content, but in cadence. After one particularly quiet session, he said, "I feel like you don't need me to be interesting." I was startled. I had never thought of him as trying to be interesting—but of course, he was. His curated self had always arrived ready for aesthetic reception, for someone to appreciate what he had shaped. But something had changed. He was no longer performing for that gaze. He had sensed my presence not as evaluative, but as rhythmic. He no longer had to fill the space. He could begin to *inhabit it*.

If the false self provides a scaffolding for temporally ordered psychic life, what happens when the scaffolding collapses? A patient who has long relied on this structure for navigating the social world may find himself unmoored in moments of rupture or affective flooding, where the ordinary rhythms of time falter. Clinical experience suggests that these moments are not experienced as dramatic or cataclysmic from the outside, but are often marked by a subtle but suffocating stillness. The patient may appear flat or compliant, but internally feels trapped in a timeless, spaceless zone—a state of psychic suspension where nothing new can happen. Here, the collapse of the false self does not disclose an authentic or spontaneous self waiting beneath, but a temporal void.

Winnicott's (1965) description of the false self was never merely a denunciation of inauthenticity; it was a developmental account of psychic survival. Yet too often, the collapse of the false self has been misread as a hopeful shedding of artifice, akin to the romantic ideal of a buried "true self" finally emerging. In clinical reality, this collapse more frequently yields a dissociative stasis, what Bollas (1987) might call an "unthought known," now unheld and unholding. The curated temporality of the false self—its capacity to sustain sequencing, delay, performative coherence—disintegrates. What replaces it is not spontaneity, but blankness.

This state of blankness often carries a hidden structure. Drawing on Eigen's (2004) concept of the "dead spot," we can understand the collapsed false self not as emptiness, but as an organized disorganization—a self-fragment attempting to preserve psychic life by halting it. The dead spot is not an absence of experience, but a defense against unbearable temporal flow. In this view, the patient is not unfeeling but overfull, not barren but saturated—yet the only tolerable way to endure that saturation is by suspending time itself. The flattening of affect, the atemporality of dissociation, and the compliant surface all serve to mummify the self in a kind of psychic sarcophagus. The false self collapses not into truth, but into stillness.

A clinical vignette may clarify this process. A patient, Leo, presented with a polished exterior, fluent in the therapeutic idiom of insight and mindfulness. For many months, he described his internal states with clarity and composure. Yet each session seemed to end at the threshold of some invisible frontier. He could narrate his suffering, but not feel it in the room. Then, one afternoon, Leo arrived visibly disorganized—distracted, irritable, and forgetful. He apologized repeatedly for being "off." As we spoke, he described a vague sense that everything had become "foggy," like the world had slowed down but without relief. He couldn't recall the sequence of events that led up to this feeling, nor could he anchor his experience in any coherent frame. He said, "It's like I'm stuck inside a paused movie—everything is happening around me, but I'm not really in it."

In that moment, the collapse of his false self was palpable not in a dramatic breakdown but in the loss of temporal coherence. The analytic task was not to peel back layers to locate a hidden core, but to witness the stalled temporality with him—to sit inside the suspended frame and lend it rhythm. I found myself slowing my speech, matching his cadence, and gently structuring the narrative fragments he offered. The goal was not to reassert the false self but to help metabolize the overwhelming sense of timeless collapse—to reintroduce the possibility of sequence, pacing, and relational time.

This clinical moment illustrates a paradox central to the false self phenomenon: its collapse is not inherently liberatory. Rather than unveiling a true self, it often reveals the scaffolding that time itself had provided. When that scaffolding is stripped away, what remains is not revelation but disorientation. The analyst's role becomes not just interpretive but rhythmic—to help the patient feel time again, from the inside.

In the next section, we will examine how some patients defensively recruit the false self precisely to avoid this collapse—employing curatorial strategies not to deceive, but to stave off an encroaching atemporality that threatens psychic dissolution.

If timeless collapse marks the failure of the false self to sustain a livable temporality, then the persistence of curatorial strategies can be understood not merely as defensive self-deception but as a desperate act of temporal preservation. Many patients unconsciously recruit their false self to fend off a feared return to the void of timelessness—to ensure that something, anything, continues to happen. This is especially evident in what might be called *curated liveliness*: a form of performative vitality that simulates spontaneity while actually functioning to preserve temporal structure and fend off psychic paralysis.

A young adult patient, Caleb, illustrates this mechanism. He arrived at treatment stylish, charismatic, and intellectually fluent—articulating a rich internal world with theatrical flair. Yet there was an uncanny sameness to his disclosures, as if each narrative had been rehearsed. Caleb would often remark, "I want to surprise myself," or "I wish I could just be more real," voicing a longing for spontaneity while compulsively preparing for it. At one point, he confessed, "Sometimes I rehearse therapy in my head so I don't waste your time." It became clear that spontaneity, for Caleb, had become a burden he could never authentically lift. The performance of surprise had replaced the experience of it.

Rather than dismantling this curated self, the analytic task was to honor its function: it was keeping time from dissolving. Caleb's false self was not shielding a hidden true self but protecting against an inner fragmentation too chaotic to narrate. This was a kind of *temporal holding*, a personal mythmaking that kept the self marginally coherent. The performance was a metronome, not a mask.

In such cases, the false self acts as a curator of temporal continuity. Drawing on Loewald (1978a), we might say that the patient's sense of sequence—past, present, future—is being held together through this performative ego. It is not deception, but substitution: instead of feeling real, the patient maintains a rhythm that simulates being alive. Without it, psychic time would collapse inward.

In the next section, we will turn toward the implications of this phenomenon for the analyst's temporality. How does the analyst's capacity to hold, pace, and even disrupt time shape the analytic pair's ability to metabolize false self structures that no longer hold?

The Analyst's Time: Holding, Disruption, and Rhythmic Encounter

If the false self curates time to keep the psyche from falling into collapse, then the analyst's temporality becomes central to the analytic process. More than an interpretive stance, the analyst's rhythm—how they speak, wait, interrupt, and return—can anchor the disorganized or frozen subject in the possibility of shared temporality. Just as a traumatized infant requires a caregiver's regulation to organize affect, the dissociative or over-curated adult may rely on the analyst to lend rhythm, rupture, or elasticity to time.

This is not merely metaphorical. In sessions with patients whose false selves dominate, the analyst often feels a kind of internal pacing pressure: to match, modulate, or disrupt the patient's tempo. One patient's flattened affect may elicit a creeping stillness in the analyst, while another's curated sparkle may evoke a sense of being cast in a play. The countertransference is not simply emotional—it is temporal. These reactions can indicate the analyst's internal registration of the patient's disrupted or overdetermined sense of time, and may require the analyst to tune into their own embodied temporality as a clinical instrument.

Winnicott's (1965) insight that the analyst provides an environment, not just an interpretation, is especially relevant here. The analyst's temporal behavior becomes part of that holding environment. What tone, what delay, what kind of silence is being offered? When a patient collapses into timelessness, the analyst may become a temporal surrogate, sustaining a beat when the patient cannot. The analyst's presence becomes what Loewald (1978b) might describe as a "medium of transformation," where a shared psychic field allows archaic time to be rendered into a narratable, livable sequence.

Ogden's (1994) notion of the analytic third offers another dimension here: temporal rhythm is not merely enacted by patient or analyst individually, but is co-constructed through the intersubjective field. Disruption, hesitation, and silence are not static gaps but dynamic elements of this third space—capable of generating psychic time where none previously existed. When the analytic pair resonates, they can begin to metabolize previously frozen or overly curated experiences, restoring the sense of being in time together.

This is not always gentle. Sometimes, the most transformative interventions involve disrupting the false self's temporal rhythm. One patient, Mara, often filled the session with associative speed, jumping between ideas with impressive fluency but leaving no time to metabolize. She presented a curated spontaneity, but behind it lay a dread of silence. In one session, I interrupted—not harshly, but firmly—and asked her to pause. "What would happen if we didn't rush this?" I asked. She blinked, frozen. The room fell into an uncomfortably long silence. Then tears came. "It's too quiet in here," she said. "It's like I disappear."

My disruption had not been a rupture of safety, but a rupture of rhythm. By refusing to pace with her false self, I had introduced a different temporality—one in which her unformulated experience could begin to emerge. In that moment, she was not abandoned to the void but accompanied in it. The analyst's task is often to tolerate these ruptures of rhythm without prematurely rescuing or interpreting them—to allow new psychic time to slowly unfold, even if it first appears as dread or disorientation.

Another patient, Jeremy, arrived at treatment with urgency. "I need to move fast," he said. "I'm tired of talking about my childhood. I want to fix what's broken and get on with things." His disclosures were full of energy—intense, emotionally charged, but delivered in a rapid, compressed style. At first, I mistook this for openness. But I soon realized I was struggling to breathe in the sessions. I felt pulled into a tempo that wasn't mine—pressured to be more active, more useful, more immediate.

I began to feel that if I did not offer something soon, I would fail him. This pressure, I came to understand, was not simply a reflection of his personality, but a temporal strategy: to keep the session moving so that nothing too painful could settle. His false self wasn't polished like Mara's—it was kinetic. It demanded speed as a form of control. If we slowed down, something might erupt.

One day, midway through his rapid account of a romantic breakup, I asked, gently but deliberately, "Can we stop here for a moment?" He stiffened. "Why? We're finally getting to the point." I said, "That's exactly why." We sat in silence. He looked frustrated. But he didn't leave.

Over the next few weeks, his rhythm didn't change dramatically, but the silences became less charged. He began to tolerate not knowing. There were sessions where he allowed space between thoughts, where he asked what I thought instead of pre-empting it. The urgency softened. He told me, "Sometimes I think if I slow down, I'll lose control. But I guess I never really had it."

This moment revealed a deeper rhythm forming—not one imposed by me, but co-created. He was beginning to experiment with time as something he could inhabit rather than outrun. The analytic task was not to force stillness, but to survive the fear of it with him.

Benjamin (1995) has written of recognition as a moment of meeting—not a final knowing, but a temporal opening. In this light, the analyst's rhythm is less a technique than a mode of recognition, a way of saying: I am here, I will wait with you, we can bear this unfolding together. Rhythmic encounter, then, becomes not just a support for the patient's experience of time, but a shared act of witnessing the conditions under which time becomes possible again.

The analyst's time is not neutral. It is a temporal offering, a frame within which dissociation might soften, curated performance might be held without demand, and new rhythms of selfhood might form. To work with the false self is to work with time: how it is organized, stalled, saturated, and shared.

In the final section, we will turn toward how the false self might evolve rather than collapse—how time, when held long enough and well enough, can begin to transform the structures it once protected.

Time, Truth, and Transformation

If the false self protects the psyche through temporal curation, and its collapse threatens a timeless void, then what does it mean for the false self to evolve? Can the structures once erected in defense of psychic coherence become scaffolds for transformation? This section proposes that under sustained, rhythmic holding, the false self may undergo a quiet metamorphosis—not into a truer self hidden beneath, but into a more complex subjectivity capable of bearing layered time.

In this view, transformation is not a sudden revelation but a slow accretion. The self does not shed artifice like a mask, but integrates its functions—holding, delaying, sequencing—into a more elastic psychic form. This process resembles what Loewald (1978d) described as a move from concreteness to symbolization, where the analytic relationship fosters a temporal field in which disparate parts of the self may begin to coexist rather than collapse or compete.

Take, for instance, a patient who begins treatment with a high defensive structure: punctual, composed, and articulate, but emotionally disengaged. Over the years of analytic work, the false self may not disappear, but it becomes less rigid. The patient begins to tolerate moments of pause, contradiction, and even disarray. Affect, once sequestered behind performance, seeps into the room unbidden. When asked what has changed, the patient might say, "I don't feel like I'm performing anymore—but I also don't feel like I've become someone else. I just feel more here."

This form of change is not about discovering a hidden authenticity but about expanding the tolerable range of psychic time. The self becomes more temporally diverse: able to pause, to meander, to return. Transitional phenomena, as described by Winnicott (1953), offer a clue here. Just as the child uses a transitional object to bridge internal and external reality, the evolving false self may become a transitional structure—one that holds temporal contradiction and ambiguity rather than foreclosing them.

Ferenczi's (1933) insights into the elasticity of psychic time also resonate. His recognition that trauma can fragment temporality—leaving parts of the psyche frozen or accelerated—foreshadows the idea that healing is not merely cathartic but temporal. To transform is to re-enter time. In analysis, this means fostering a relational field in which these frozen or hurried parts can find new pacing, new sequence, and new relational rhythm.

Importantly, such transformation does not require the annihilation of the false self. Rather, it asks that we see the false self as a developmental achievement that once safeguarded the psyche and now seeks relational recontextualization. What was once rigidly curative may become creatively adaptive. In this light, the analyst's task is not to unmask the patient, but to accompany them as they reinhabit their own psychic time.

This echoes Bollas's (1987) vision of the "true self experience" not as the emergence of a hidden essence, but as a felt sense of vitality and continuity within the lived moment. What transforms, then, is not just the self, but its way of being in time.

When the false self begins to evolve, it often does so unevenly, in micro-movements. These are not dramatic unveilings but small shifts in rhythm: a pause where there used to be chatter; a sigh where once there was silence; a spontaneous memory; a shared laugh. These are moments in which psychic time becomes shared time, and the internal curator begins to soften.

The transformation of the false self is not a destination but an ongoing temporal negotiation. It marks the patient's increasing capacity to dwell in the unfinished, the in-between, the asynchronous. And it marks the analyst's willingness to join them there—not to organize or interpret too quickly, but to linger long enough that something new might form.

In this way, analysis becomes a space not simply of insight but of time restored: time that is slow, recursive, relational, and ultimately transformative. Time that can hold the self without hardening it. Time that becomes a medium of truth—not because it reveals an essence, but because it allows the self to unfold.

Epilogue: Aftertime

Not every self collapses. Some endure through choreography—repeating, curating, rehearsing life until it becomes just bearable enough to live. In the analytic room, these selves do not ask to be unveiled. They ask to be timed with. And if the analyst listens closely, what comes forward is not a secret but a sequence—a rhythm held just long enough to keep the self from shattering.

There is no final breakthrough in such work, no single moment where the false self dissolves and something more "real" steps forward. The false self does not yield to authenticity; it yields to rhythm. To accompaniment. To a temporality that no longer demands protection through performance.

This is the quiet miracle of analytic time: that a self can become more livable not through revelation, but through pacing. Through waiting. Through the shared labor of surviving unfinishedness. The analyst offers not a solution but a beat, a contour, a breath. We do not interpret our way toward truth. We co-create a rhythm in which the self can begin—cautiously, unevenly—to feel time without fearing it.

In the end, what endures is not catharsis, but continuity. Not the arrival of a true self, but the fading of urgency. The patient may still perform, still retreat, still displace. But these movements are no longer saturated with dread. They become part of a longer rhythm—recursive, human, survivable. And in that rhythm, the self may begin to unfold.

Not quickly. And never all at once.

9 The False Self as Curator

Symbolic Life, Containment, and the Paradox of Authenticity

This chapter explores the false self not as a pathological mask but as a symbolic curator—a psychic structure that mediates survival, aesthetic form, and relational hope. Drawing on Winnicott's original theory and extending it through developmental, philosophical, and queer theoretical lenses, the chapter reframes the false/true self dichotomy as a paradox to be inhabited rather than resolved. Integrating contributions from Loewald, Bollas, Chasseguet-Smirgel, Orange, Stern, Damasio, and Bromberg—as well as thinkers such as Foucault, Wittgenstein, Heidegger, and Sullivan—the argument treats the false self as an intelligent architecture shaped by misrecognition and held aliveness. Rather than seeing authenticity as the undoing of the false self, it is reframed as a relational achievement made possible by containment, performance, and symbolic resonance.

This chapter examines ego ideals and the fantasy of the true self, symbolic vitality and its regulation, secrecy and non-experience, and the false self's role in managing unsymbolized affect. Through clinical vignettes and theoretical elaboration, the false self is presented not as something to unmask, but to understand and witness. Symbolic life does not begin when performance ends; it begins when the curations of the self are received with ethical presence. The analyst's task is not to dismantle what protects but to recognize its aesthetic and survival function—until it no longer carries that burden alone.

The Paradox of the Self

The desire to live authentically presumes that somewhere, within or behind experience, a self exists that can be accessed, known, and expressed—a self not distorted by expectation, compliance, or fear. In the consulting room, this longing appears often as dissatisfaction: with performance, with relationships, with one's own sincerity. "I don't know who I am," a patient might say, not with theatrical flourish but with an aching fatigue. The phrase does not describe confusion so much as disconnection—a lived paradox in which the self is both too much and nowhere at all.

The false self emerges here not as a pathology but as a structure of meaning. It is not necessarily defensive, nor is it always deceptive. It is often a

DOI: 10.4324/9781003715283-12

necessary translation—of aliveness into legibility, of feeling into form. And yet, within the symbolic logic of psychoanalysis, to form the self is always to fracture it. Every act of representation divides the experience it seeks to carry. The paradox is not a problem to solve but the very architecture of selfhood: we become ourselves only through a recursive series of displacements.

This paradox is not new. In Winnicott's vocabulary, the distinction between true and false self was never meant as a dichotomy. The true self, he wrote, refers to spontaneity, a sense of aliveness unmediated by external demands. But this aliveness cannot appear unless there is a sufficient holding environment—a world in which the spontaneous gesture can land and be metabolized. Absent that, the false self emerges not as falsification but as accommodation. It performs stability to protect what cannot yet be expressed. And yet this performance, in time, becomes mistaken for the self itself. Winnicott's greatest insight may have been his ambivalence: that the false self may carry vitality, too, that compliance can be creative, and that what looks like artifice may in fact be survival.

The foundational split—between what is lived and what is shown—is not merely developmental. It is ontological. *There is no true self without form, but the moment the self takes form, it has been altered.* This is the recursive impossibility upon which the self is built. In the earlier chapter, *The Original Paradox*, I described this as the foundational rhythm of psychic life: a looping structure in which fragmentation does not signal failure but returns as structure, symbol, even gesture. That insight echoes here. The false self is not the opposite of the real, but its only possible medium.

Theoretical traditions have named this split differently. **Loewald** speaks of internalization as the process that transforms the primitive into the symbolic. For him, the self is not discovered but *formed* in and through the symbolic field. **Wittgenstein**, from a different lens, reminds us that the most essential aspects of life cannot be *said*, only *shown*. This difference—between what can be articulated and what must be enacted—haunts every attempt to live authentically. The self must be performed in order to be seen, but the performance never quite matches the feeling. The paradox persists: we show ourselves in ways that distort us, and we hide in order to be found.

Heidegger adds a further complication. His notion of *thrownness*—that we are always already situated in a world not of our choosing—undermines the fantasy of a self untouched by context. The true self, then, cannot be prior to adaptation. It is always emerging, always entangled, always formed under conditions of contingency. Even our most inward longings are shaped by histories not fully ours. If Winnicott emphasized the developmental holding environment, Heidegger gives us the ontological field—the *being-with* that structures all experience.

This raises a further paradox. If the true self is imagined as untouched, spontaneous, essential—and the false self as responsive, curated, contingent—then we must ask: *where do we locate meaning?* Is authenticity a matter of impulse or of responsibility? Can the curated self not also carry vitality, symbolization, and care?

The **ego ideal**, as Freud conceived it, complicates things even further. It is the internalized observer, the self one wishes to become, or imagines one should already be. It regulates, judges, inspires, and accuses. Often, in patients struggling with identity, it is the ego ideal—not the external world—that generates the most punishing anxiety. "I should feel more," one patient says. "I should be realer." The ego ideal, in these cases, often masquerades as the true self: an unachievable standard, projected into the psyche as both a moral imperative and aesthetic demand.

This patient, for instance—a man in his early 30s—had spent his entire adolescence perfecting what he called his "invisible self." There was no trauma in the usual sense, only an atmosphere of evaluation so pervasive that even his pleasures had become performances. He could express emotion convincingly, even tenderly, but afterward would report feeling empty—as if the feeling had been something he did rather than something that passed through him. "Even when I cry," he told me, "it feels like I'm doing it for someone else." The self he longed for was not simply more real—it was impossible. It was a self untethered from audience, unformed by context, unsplit by expectation. What he had instead—and what we came to respect—was a self that had learned how to be legible, how to survive, how to perform sincerity so well it nearly became truth. He did not need to discard this structure, but to find within it a place to rest.

Chasseguet-Smirgel would remind us that the ego ideal, while necessary for development, easily tips into perversion—not sexual, but symbolic. It distorts growth into mimicry and desire into compliance. And yet, like the false self, it carries the trace of hope. The self that wishes to become is a self that is still alive. The tragedy lies not in the longing but in mistaking the ideal for something that must already be achieved.

Harry Stack Sullivan reminds us that the self is not a static structure but a "reflected appraisals" process—formed in and through relationships, always shifting, contingent, and field-dependent. This supports what Winnicott already knew: that the capacity to be alone is not the absence of others, but the internalization of a reliable other's presence. The paradox of aloneness—that we are only alone when we are sufficiently held—mirrors the paradox of the self: that we can only become ourselves through the forms we internalize, repeat, and curate. The false self, in this reading, is not a deviation from the real, but its earliest architecture.

What follows in this chapter will take these contradictions seriously. Rather than dividing the self into good and bad, authentic and false, we will consider the false self as a symbolic structure—a curator of thresholds, an aesthetic strategy, a holding form. This requires relinquishing the fantasy of undistorted *being* and instead embracing what Orange has called "empathic co-construction"—the relational shaping of what is livable. The false self is not the failure of authenticity. It is its precondition.

Winnicott's False Self System: Ambivalence, Adaptation, and Survival

Winnicott's theory of the false self has become so culturally absorbed—so intuitively resonant—that it often risks being flattened into a cliché: the idea that one must discard artifice to uncover a purer self beneath. But Winnicott himself was far less moralistic. His descriptions of the false self are ambivalent, layered, and saturated with clinical humility. He did not condemn it—he studied its functions. He did not idealize the true self—he knew how fragile it could be.

In his paper, *Ego Distortion in Terms of True and False Self*, Winnicott (1965) lays out a spectrum of false self formations, ranging from adaptive and creative to empty and deadened. At the healthiest end, the false self is a polite facade—a necessary interface with the world, preserving the privacy of deeper experience. At the most compromised end, the false self becomes a total substitute, hollowing out spontaneity and leaving the subject uncertain that any internal experience is truly their own. But what makes his account radical is the refusal to condemn the false self. It is not the enemy of authenticity, but its container—a defensive but often creative response to failures of early recognition.

The origins of the false self, for Winnicott, lie in the *environmental failure* of infancy—particularly the failure of maternal attunement. If the environment cannot tolerate the infant's spontaneous gestures, the infant adapts. The false self forms not because the infant wants to deceive, but because the infant must preserve some contact—any contact—with the caregiver. It is, in this sense, a tragic compromise: protecting the core self through mimicry, attunement through surrender, aliveness through performance. And in time, if the false self is never softened or witnessed, it becomes not a layer but a prison.

And yet Winnicott does not leave us there. In his work, there is a quiet confidence that the false self remains tethered to the real. Even the most defended patients can produce a gesture—a flicker of spontaneity—that feels alive. When this happens in the therapeutic relationship, it is not dramatic. It is often subtle: a moment of quiet that is not empty, a joke that is not practiced, a look that does not retreat. These are not eruptions of the true self but gestures of *possibility*—signs that the false self is not a tomb but a membrane.

Winnicott's theory is shaped by his own clinical and historical context. Writing in the decades following World War II, Winnicott had witnessed the psychic damage caused not just by trauma but by silence, by absence, by rupture in early care. Unlike Klein, who focused on internal object relations and phantasy life, Winnicott looked outward—to the environment, to the holding conditions of early development. He understood that the ego does not form in isolation. It forms in relation to whether or not one's gestures land.

This emphasis on environment is most powerfully seen in his concept of the *holding environment*—a phrase now ubiquitous but often under-theorized. For Winnicott, holding is not simply physical but emotional, symbolic, and temporal. It is the reliable, attuned, not-too-intrusive presence that allows the infant to begin believing in their own existence. When holding fails, the infant does not protest—they adapt. And this adaptation, while often brilliant, can be costly. The self that performs well is not always the self that feels.

The paradox continues in his essay *The Capacity to Be Alone*. Winnicott's central argument is itself a provocation: the ability to be alone is not innate—it must be developed, and only in the presence of a non-intrusive, reliably available other. This is not simply a developmental claim but a philosophical one. Even aloneness, which we imagine as the domain of the true self, is founded on relational presence. To be alone is always to be *alone with someone*. The false self—so often cast as a barrier—may in fact be the only structure within which a patient can risk aloneness. It protects not just against intrusion but against collapse.

Masud Khan, Winnicott's patient, student, and eventual collaborator, also contributed to this tension. While Khan's personal and professional ethics were ultimately discredited, his clinical writing on self-deception, fragmentation, and the protective function of the false self remains relevant. He extended Winnicott's ideas to the analytic field, suggesting that the false self was not merely historical but actively shaped in the relational environment of the session. The analyst's attunement—or lack thereof—continues the early conditions that either permit or prevent contact with the real.

Here, the false self becomes less a developmental stage and more a **symbolic strategy**—a way of managing the potential rupture of misrecognition. In clinical work, this often means respecting the false self as a *living structure*, not a mask to be ripped away. One must learn to speak through it, to listen beneath it, to tolerate its necessity. Premature interpretations that attempt to expose the "real" can collapse the field. Often, the analyst must wait, bearing the muted frustration that comes with curated engagement, before the self begins to risk aliveness.

Consider a patient who describes every emotion with precision, fluency, and even poetic grace—and yet never seems moved. They narrate their interiority with perfect insight, but there is no friction, no mess, no surprise. Every expression is buffered, buffered again, and offered like a gift wrapped twice. At first, the analyst may be seduced: this is a "good patient," someone who can think, reflect, and verbalize. However, over time, it becomes clear that what is being shared is not the experience itself, but rather a representation. The false self, here, is not a performance in the theatrical sense—it is a *containment strategy*, designed not to deceive but to protect. The analyst must ask not, "What are you hiding?" but "What happens if this stops working?"

In these cases, Winnicott's insight is invaluable: what is feared is not exposure, but collapse. The false self protects not against being known but against being unheld. Its task is not concealment but *coherence*—to maintain the illusion of symbolic continuity when the inner world feels too unformed to risk contact. The analyst's job is not to dismantle it, but to offer a new kind of holding—one that allows experience to become thinkable, feelable, survivable.

Harry Stack Sullivan's interpersonal theory supports this stance. For Sullivan, the self is not an entity but a pattern—a set of reflected appraisals and interactions that solidify over time. There is no essential core, no autonomous authenticity, only an evolving field of responses to anxiety, safety, and recognition. In this light, the false self is not the opposite of the real—it is the self, structured around the field in which it was formed.

And yet, even Sullivan's fluidity benefits from Winnicott's tenderness. For Winnicott, there is still something—not essential, but **longing**. Something in the patient that reaches for unmediated contact, that aches to be held without adapting. The false self is not a refusal of this longing. It is its expression—in code, in caution, in the syntax of safety.

The Ego Ideal and the Fiction of the "True" Self

The notion of a "true self" often circulates in the cultural imagination as a kind of latent purity—a hidden essence waiting to be uncovered, expressed, and finally lived. In therapy, this idea emerges frequently in language saturated with longing: "I want to feel like myself again," or "I just want to be real." These statements are rarely about specific memories or identities; they refer instead to a self imagined as coherent, spontaneous, and emotionally congruent. But as psychoanalysis has long recognized, the idea of the "true self" is itself a symbolic construction—one closely bound to the **ego ideal**.

Freud introduced the ego ideal in his 1914 paper *On Narcissism*, distinguishing it from both the ego and the superego. The ego ideal, he proposed, is the internalized image of the self one wishes to become—a psychic heir to early experiences of being idealized by others. In infancy, when the self is first mirrored, the parent's gaze confers not just recognition but grandeur. The child feels omnipotent, central, and radiant. As development progresses, this early fusion fractures, and the child begins to internalize both the idealized parental gaze and the standard to which they must now aspire. The ego ideal becomes the new audience—internal, unrelenting, both exalted and exacting.

Over time, this internal observer—once protective—can become tyrannical. In many patients, the ego ideal operates not as a source of aspiration but as a source of shame. "I should be more present," "I should be more open," "I should feel more." The longing to be "real" is frequently a disguised demand issued by the ego ideal itself—a demand to reach a state of undistorted, perfectly congruent experience. Ironically, this imagined "true self" is often more rigid and less compassionate than the false self it seeks to replace.

In her work on creativity and perversion, Chasseguet-Smirgel emphasizes that the ego ideal, when overdeveloped, can arrest development. The subject no longer seeks to grow through symbolization but to return to an imagined state of perfection. Idealization collapses into omnipotence; aspiration becomes a refusal of limitation. In this light, the pursuit of the true self can become a perverse fantasy—again, not in the sexual sense, but in the structural sense: a defense against fragmentation, vulnerability, and contradiction.

Yet the ego ideal is not simply a pathology. As Loewald suggests, it also serves as a developmental horizon—a symbolic structure that allows the subject to imagine transformation. It is the self-in-becoming, the space between who I am and who I might be. In therapy, when a patient begins to differentiate the ego ideal from the ego—begins to grieve the fantasy and tolerate symbolic imperfection—something vital shifts. They do not discard the ideal, but they relate to it differently. It becomes a guide, not a tyrant. The goal is no longer to become perfect, but to live symbolically—to hold contradiction without collapse.

Still, the fiction of the true self lingers, especially in those who feel they have performed too long. A queer patient once described the process of "coming out" not as revelation but as collapse. "I had spent so many years imagining that there was a real me trapped under all the performance," he said. "But when I tried to live as that person, I realized he didn't exist. I had no idea what I actually wanted. I only knew how to want things for other people." What he experienced was not the emergence of the true self, but the shattering of the ego ideal. The self he had imagined as latent turned out to be a construction, and when it failed to materialize, he felt abandoned by it. He had mistaken the ideal for the real, and when the ideal dissolved, he was left not with authenticity but with emptiness.

Tim Dean, writing from a queer psychoanalytic perspective, explores this phenomenon with striking clarity. He argues that much of gay shame stems not simply from marginalization but from the **internalization of impossible standards of psychic coherence**—the demand to be legible, sincere, and integrated. For Dean, the queer subject often finds himself structured by the fantasy of "becoming whole," a fantasy that is not only unattainable but also anti-queer in its refusal of fragmentation. The ego ideal, in this framework, does not merely regulate desire—it imposes a normative image of selfhood that erases contradiction. The so-called "true self" is thus not a refuge, but a mirage.

Heidegger, too, is useful here. His critique of inauthenticity is not an endorsement of some pre-social essence but a recognition of the ways in which *Dasein*—the mode of human being—is always already embedded in the world, always already shaped by history, culture, and thrownness. Authenticity, for Heidegger, is not purity but engagement—a willingness to take up one's situation as one's own. In this light, the false self is not a problem to solve, but a condition to work within. The question is not "how do I become real?" but "how do I relate to my thrownness with responsibility and care?"

From this perspective, the true self is not the origin point but the remainder—what survives, what recurs, what resists full articulation. **Wittgenstein** might say that the true self is not something that can be stated, but only shown. It is not content but a gesture. Not a fixed identity but a pattern of returns. This reframing enables a more generous approach to the curated self. The question becomes not whether it is real, but whether it is *livable*—whether it can hold vitality, bear contradiction, and make room for symbolization.

Even the most performative false selves carry fragments of this longing. A patient who arrives in a carefully managed tone and gesture, always composed, rarely touched—may still, in a single unscripted moment, betray something raw. Not in the sense of rupture, but in the sense of slippage — a laugh, a silence, a sudden loss of coherence. These moments are not revelations of truth but gestures toward it. They are not eruptions of the real self, but tiny failures of the ideal—and thus, openings.

In this chapter, and those that follow, we will continue to unhook the language of authenticity from the fantasy of essence. The false self is not what we must escape to find the real. It is what we must understand, respect, and symbolically inhabit. The ego ideal, when softened, can become a horizon rather than a cage. And the true self—if it exists at all—may be the part of us that still believes there is something worth curating.

Vitality and the Curated Self

If the false self is typically framed in terms of performance, compliance, and repression, its relationship to vitality is often overlooked or misunderstood. We tend to assume that aliveness is the exclusive domain of the "true self," and that the false self, by contrast, is deadened, flat, or emotionally inert. But this dichotomy collapses under clinical scrutiny. Many patients bring highly curated selves that feel vibrantly animated—organized not by deadness but by intensity, elegance, and control. What appears constricted may in fact be pulsing with effort: a structure built to contain too much, not too little.

Vitality, as Daniel Stern articulated it, is not a single affect but a quality of experience—a kinetic signature, a sense of movement, emergence, and integration. He called these "vitality affects"—distinct from discrete emotions like anger or joy. They describe the way feeling takes form, the way the body organizes around becoming itself. Stern's work reminds us that the opposite of vitality is not numbness, but collapse. The curated self, in this view, is not necessarily lifeless. It may be the only available means of preserving aliveness in an environment where spontaneity was met with disapproval, confusion, or threat.

This is especially true in patients with developmental trauma or chronic misattunement. For them, vitality is often felt not as pleasure, but as exposure. The body quickens, the voice tightens, and something unbearable begins to flicker at the edge of consciousness. In these moments, the false self emerges as a *regulator of affective amplitude*—not to suppress life, but to keep it survivable. This dynamic frequently appears in patients who are hyper-competent, aesthetically attuned, or intellectually gifted. They live by form. Expression is not discouraged but stylized. Intensity is permitted, but only within symbolic or aesthetic contexts. They feel alive when performing—and yet afterward, they often feel emptied. The performance, while vital, is not metabolized.

One such patient, a visual artist in his late thirties, described his exhibitions as "the only times I know I'm real." During shows, he would feel a rush of contact—being seen, being understood—but afterward, a profound estrangement would set in. "It's like I disappear the moment the lights go off," he said. "The only version of me anyone wants is the one that's curated." In therapy, he initially repeated this dynamic: intensely expressive sessions followed by withdrawal, self-criticism, and doubt. His false self was not a rigid persona but an aesthetic system—intricate, intelligent, and profoundly lonely.

Antonio Damasio, working from the perspective of affective neuroscience, writes that the sense of self is not an abstract concept but a continuously generated mapping of bodily states—a felt narrative of survival. When emotional experience threatens coherence, the system constricts. This is not repression in the Freudian sense, but a modulation of the organism's need to endure. In this light, the false self can be seen as a *bodily defense against psychic flooding*. Its task is not to deaden, but to buffer. What looks like affective flatness may actually be a saturated container—one whose walls must hold tightly to preserve its function.

This challenges the notion that therapeutic work should aim to dismantle the false self in pursuit of emotional "truth." For many patients, emotional truth—unfiltered, unsymbolized—would be psychically disorganizing. What they need is not liberation from structure, but a new kind of symbolic space in which vitality can be titrated. Here, the analyst must tread carefully. When the patient begins to feel more—more desire, more pain, more spontaneity—they may also begin to panic. The self that has spent years managing expression now risks unraveling. Vitality is not always welcome.

Donna Orange, in her work on witnessing and emotional understanding, emphasizes that vitality requires not just space, but relationship. Aliveness becomes livable only when it is seen and held. It is not enough to "feel more." One must feel with. This is particularly important in the treatment of dissociative structures, where affective intensities often emerge unformulated and overwhelming. The false self, in these cases, is a *scaffold for experience that has not yet been borne*. It allows time, metaphor, rhythm—the conditions in which symbolization might occur.

In therapy, this process can be slow and often imperceptible. A patient may begin to speak with less precision, pause more often, and allow uncertainty to enter the room. These changes are not signs of breakdown but of *loosening containment*. The curated self becomes less necessary when the therapeutic environment offers a more responsive holding. But this is not a linear progression. Often, as soon as spontaneity emerges, the false self reasserts itself—refining, translating, restoring coherence. This is not regression, but rather survival. The analyst must not demand vulnerability too soon. Instead, they must *trust the aesthetic intelligence of the false self*—its ability to signal, in stylized form, what cannot yet be spoken.

Christopher Bollas offers a resonant concept here: the *unthought known*. These are experiences that have shaped us deeply but were never verbalized—never symbolically formulated. They live in the body, the tone of voice, and the rhythm of speech. The false self is often the custodian of these experiences. It holds what cannot yet be remembered. In this way, it becomes not a lie, but a latency—a form of future expression.

This recasts the question of authenticity. Instead of asking whether a moment is "real," we might ask whether it carries **symbolic vitality**—whether it emerges from the patient's own rhythm, not in defiance of containment, but within it. The curated self, at its most flexible, allows for this. It does not erase the self but stages it. It makes performance a form of practice—a space to try on aliveness before it becomes lived reality.

To be clear, this is not an argument against spontaneity. Rather, it is an argument against the moralization of it. In many analytic traditions, there remains a subtle bias in favor of the raw, the unrehearsed, the primal. But for many patients—especially queer, neurodivergent, or developmentally complex patients—spontaneity is not a sign of health. It is a risk. Their selves have been organized around the need to manage, to stage, to stylize. These are not neuroses to be undone, but **aesthetic systems** to be respected, interpreted, and sometimes softened.

The goal is not to destroy the false self, but to find vitality within it. To listen not just to what it hides, but to what it knows. The curated self may hold the patient's deepest longings—in code, in gesture, in form. It may be the only part of the self brave enough to appear. And when it does, the analyst's task is not to expose it, but to accompany it—until, perhaps, it no longer needs to carry so much alone.

The False Self as Curator

The metaphor of the false self as a *mask* has long shaped both clinical thinking and cultural narratives. It suggests deception, concealment, a performance put on to hide what is "real." But this image fails to capture the nuance and complexity of the curated self. Not all masks are lies. Some are scaffolds. Some are offerings. Some are the only way a self dares to appear. The false self is less a disguise than a *curatorial act*—a structure of psychic design that protects, arranges, and filters relational contact in a world that may not yet be able to hold the unscripted.

To think of the false self as a *curator* is to shift the analytic gaze from exposure to architecture. A curator does not create the artwork but selects and frames it. She tends to context, invites legibility, and mediates between the interior and the audience. The false self operates similarly. It assembles a version of the self that can circulate—that can function, relate, perform—while protecting what is not yet metabolized. And like any act of curation, it reflects both constraint and aesthetic intelligence.

This is not to romanticize the false self. Many patients live within it as if it were a museum with no back rooms—all display, no privacy. Others treat it as a gallery they themselves cannot access, presenting an image of liveliness while feeling profoundly alienated. But even here, the curatorial metaphor helps. It reminds us that these structures were not chosen arbitrarily. They were *often designed, and sometimes* brilliantly, to meet environmental demands. And they continue to serve—even if the cost has become unbearable.

The cultural imperative toward "authenticity"—to "be yourself," to "drop the act"—often reinforces shame in patients whose very survival has depended on the act. But what if the act is also the only portal to connection? Adam Phillips, writing on secrecy and sincerity, notes that "we speak not only to reveal ourselves but to conceal ourselves." The self is never wholly given. Every act of speech—even confession—is already shaped for an internal or imagined audience. In this light, the curated self is not a problem to be solved, but a condition to be understood.

In queer lives especially, curation is a familiar practice. Eve Sedgwick's writing on the closet offers not just a metaphor but a structure: secrecy as survival, legibility as risk. The curated self is not a deviation from truth but a navigation of exposure. The closet is not merely a space of hiding; it is also a space of *arranging*—of deciding what is shown, when, and to whom. José Muñoz elaborates on this in his work on queer futurity: performance, he argues, is not the opposite of truth but its anticipation. The self performed today may become real tomorrow. The false self becomes the site of potential—a rehearsal space for selves not yet permitted to arrive.

Ann Pellegrini furthers this line of thought by reminding us that performance is always racialized, gendered, and historically situated. What looks like curation in one subject may be read as deception in another—depending on social legibility and power. For many patients, the false self is not merely a psychic structure but a political necessity. The ability to perform well—to manage affect, to present safety—is often the condition of survival. And yet, this same performance can leave the subject estranged from the very vitality it is meant to protect.

Michel Foucault helps us reframe this further. His work on confession and surveillance in *The History of Sexuality* shows how power demands visibility. The self is not just performed—it is produced under discursive and institutional pressure. In this sense, the curated self is not only self-imposed; it is co-created by the gaze that demands it. For patients shaped by systems of control—families, schools, clinical settings—the curated self may be the only acceptable form the self can take. It is not a mask over the truth, but the only way truth is permitted to appear.

One patient, a young Black woman training to be a therapist, described how exhausting it was to be "the good one"—always composed, always prepared, always the voice of calm. She did not speak of this identity with pride but with fatigue. "If I show up messy, I lose credibility," she said. "If I don't perform it, no one believes I'm okay. But if I do, they stop asking." Her false self was not chosen—it was required. In therapy, she began to test the possibility of fragmentation: not a collapse, but a rebalancing. The curated self did not disappear, but it became more porous. Sometimes it even stepped aside.

In these moments, the false self does not dissolve. It softens. It becomes less defensive, more flexible. It allows what Loewald might call a *transformation of internalization*: the symbolic possibility that the self can become something new without the total loss of continuity. The analyst's task here is not to strip away the curatorial frame but to enter into it—to speak to the part of the patient that *chose* this form, that arranged this architecture. Interpretation may come, but only after attunement.

This is especially true in cases where the false self carries **aesthetic coherence**. Some patients bring a curated presence that is not simply performative but beautiful—carefully tended, even elegant. Their clothes, syntax, affect, and silences form a whole. To dismantle this structure would be a violation. The analyst must begin with reverence: not to idealize the false self, but to respect its role as both defense and expression.

In many ways, this mirrors the **holding function** of the analytic frame. The frame itself is a kind of curated structure—a ritualized form that contains emotion, conflict, and risk. We do not consider the frame false. We recognize it as a condition of truth-telling. The false self operates similarly. It is the patient's self-generated frame—often rigid, but sometimes capable of holding new experience. The analyst who respects this function can work within it. Those who try to dismantle it too quickly will encounter rupture.

There is a temptation to seek the "real" patient beneath the curated surface—to wait for a slip, a disclosure, a moment of affective mess that feels more "authentic." But the curated self is not necessarily hiding something. It may be offering the very best it can. The performance itself may be the site of intimacy. In such moments, the analyst must risk presence without interpretation—to accompany rather than excavate.

Winnicott knew this. His ambivalence toward the false self reflects a deep respect for the symbolic function of survival. The patient who performs well may not be faking. They may be surviving with great care. And survival is not a failure of the self. It is its first act of meaning-making.

The metaphor of curation allows us to see the false self not as a fixed persona, but as a symbolic strategy—one that filters experience, protects aliveness, and negotiates recognition. Like any good curator, the false self is working with limited resources. It arranges. It protects. It communicates. And sometimes, when it is met with care, it changes.

Mutual Dependency of True and False Selves

The temptation to separate the "true" self from the "false" self—to imagine one as essential and the other as performative—runs deep in both psychoanalytic and cultural discourse. It offers a comforting fantasy: that beneath the layers of compliance and adaptation lies a self untouched by compromise. But in Winnicott's more subtle writings, and in clinical experience more broadly, what emerges is a more complicated truth: **true and false selves are not fixed entities, but relational positions**—recursive structures of expression, defense, and longing that arise in response to holding and misrecognition.

In many patients, especially those with histories of developmental trauma, the false self has become so entrenched that the "real" self is difficult to locate. Yet something appears—a flicker of affect, a tone shift, a hesitancy that surprises both analyst and patient. These are not eruptions of authenticity but glimpses of **symbolic play**—moments when the false self becomes flexible enough to allow emergence without collapse. The true self, in such cases, does not arrive fully formed. It is not a rediscovery but a *co-creation*, born in the space between defenses and recognition.

Winnicott himself hints at this in his statement that the false self "defends the true self, which is hidden." This is often read as a hierarchy—one self protecting the other—but it may be more accurate to read it as a **relational sequence**. The false self develops in response to environmental failure. The true self retreats, not because it is weak, but because it lacks a frame. What survives is the adaptation. And that adaptation becomes the medium through which the true self might one day reappear.

But there is no return. The true self is not a prelapsarian state to be reclaimed. It is always shaped by the false self's negotiations. It grows through the gaps, the failures, the curated gestures that didn't quite succeed. In this sense, the **false self becomes the matrix of symbolic possibility**—the scaffolding through which the self might begin to live symbolically, not just protectively.

Philip Bromberg's theory of multiple self-states expands this view. For Bromberg, the self is never singular but comprised of dissociative configurations—each with its own history, affect, and internal logic. Health does not mean integration into one coherent self, but the capacity to "stand in the spaces" between these states without collapse. This capacity allows for **movement**, **metaphor**, and **symbolization**—the conditions of psychic vitality. The false self, in this frame, is one state among many. It may dominate when safety is at stake, but it is not the whole self. Nor is the true self. Both are relational postures—patterned responses to internal and external fields.

This has profound implications for clinical work. When the analyst joins with the patient in the pursuit of the "true self," there is often an unconscious rejection of the false one. The analyst longs for spontaneity, rupture, emotional immediacy—imagining that only then will the real work begin. But this longing, while understandable, can easily re-enact the very misrecognition that first necessitated the false self. The patient's curated structure is not simply a defense. It is also a **bid**—an attempt to relate on terms that feel survivable. When the analyst respects this offering, the frame becomes expansive. When they reject it, the space contracts.

This does not mean avoiding interpretation or remaining passive. It means listening to the false self as a symbolic language. What is being communicated by the perfection, the silence, the control? What kind of affect is being shaped or displayed? What threshold is being managed? The false self often signals its own limits. It shows when it is struggling to contain what lies beneath. These moments are fragile. If handled with attunement, they become openings. If rushed, they collapse.

In one session, a patient known for his self-discipline and verbal fluency paused mid-sentence. He had been describing a moment of conflict at work—narrating it with elegance, insight, and precision—when suddenly, he stopped. "I'm telling you what happened," he said, "but I don't know if I felt any of it." The room shifted. It was not a dramatic rupture, but a **questioning of curation**. His false self was not abandoned—it remained—but it made space for doubt. For Winnicott, this would be a moment of potential: not the appearance of the true self, but the first sign that the curated one no longer needs to carry everything alone.

Donna Orange's work on mutual recognition is crucial here. She reframes authenticity not as an individual achievement but as a **relational capacity**. The self becomes more real not by uncovering its essence, but by finding itself in the eyes of another who can hold contradiction. The analyst's job is not to name the true self but to make space for it—to allow its partial, hesitant, and symbolic forms to emerge and be met.

The process is recursive. The more the false self is held without contempt, the more it can soften. And the more it softens, the more something else appears—not purer, but more *alive*. That aliveness, paradoxically, may still pass through the false self. It may be stylized, curated, or tentative. That does not make it false. It makes it **symbolic**. And symbolization is the currency of psychic life.

The fantasy of full authenticity—a moment in which the self is fully seen, fully expressed, fully received—is powerful but dangerous. It often reproduces the ego ideal's demand for coherence. The analyst must be cautious not to collude with this fantasy. The goal is not to arrive at the true self, but to foster the patient's ability to **move among selves**, to tolerate contradiction, and to live within structures that are flexible enough to carry vitality.

This requires attention not only to content but to **form**. How does the patient speak? What rhythms, hesitations, and repetitions shape the session? Often, the patient's false self can be felt in the way speech is held together—in the careful syntax, the precision of language, the pauses that avoid rupture. The analyst's listening must attune to these patterns not to disrupt them, but to understand them. Interpretation, when it comes, must speak to the *aesthetic logic* of the self—the way it has been composed.

Heidegger, again, is useful here. His notion of authenticity is not about discovering the self, but about owning one's thrownness—living deliberately within the context one did not choose. The curated self, in this light, is not a betrayal of being, but a response to it. The work of therapy is not to discard the curation, but to enter it—to dwell in it with the patient until it becomes less of a shelter and more of a space.

The true self and false self are not adversaries. They are **co-constitutive**, born together in the crucible of early experience. The false self guards, arranges, and survives. The true self appears when the conditions are right—not as essence, but as expression. And often, it needs the false self to make its arrival tolerable.

To stand in the paradox is the work. The analyst holds the space where contradiction is not pathology, but rather a structure. The patient learns not to reject the curated self, but to relate to it. To listen to what it knows, what it fears, what it has held. In this way, the analytic relationship becomes a new kind of container—one in which the self is not discovered, but assembled.

Secrecy, Non-Experience, and the Fear of Breakdown

In his 1974 paper *Fear of Breakdown*, Winnicott proposed one of his most quietly radical ideas: that what the patient fears has already occurred. The breakdown is not impending—it is remembered without having been experienced. It was lived through without containment and survived without symbolization. This fear, Winnicott argued, is the echo of an absence—not a discrete trauma, but the failure of a holding environment to metabolize experience. In this way, the psyche stores not only memory but also non-experience—events that could not be borne and thus remain unformed.

The false self emerges in this context as a structure designed not to deceive, but to protect. It arranges psychic life in a way that avoids triggering what was once uncontainable. The self is curated not only for social legibility but for internal coherence. The analyst who interprets too quickly, who insists on the immediacy of emotional truth, may inadvertently force an encounter with a breakdown the patient is not yet symbolically equipped to experience.

Secrecy plays a crucial role in this architecture. It is often associated with avoidance or repression, but as Christopher Bollas reminds us, secrecy is also a form of care. It preserves what is not yet thinkable. The false self is the steward of these secrets—not because the truth is shameful, but because the symbolic apparatus for receiving it has not yet been built. The patient may speak of nothing, or everything, or in tangents that seem unrelated. But the rhythm, the gaps, the repetitions—these are part of a hidden grammar. The analyst must learn to listen not only for what is said, but for the **symbolic signature of non-experience**.

This listening requires a particular kind of presence—one attuned not to content but to atmosphere. Michael Eigen, writing on secrecy and the psychotic core, describes these spaces as thick with unsymbolized affect. The patient may dissociate, become vague, or suddenly shift tone. These are not defenses in the classical sense. They are *residues of what could not be metabolized*. In such moments, the false self does not block access to the real. It absorbs the real on the patient's behalf. It survives in the place of the self that could not yet speak.

One queer patient, in his fifties, arrived in treatment after decades of high-functioning professionalism. His life was marked by curation: polished speech, aesthetic precision, relational control. He spoke openly about being gay, about his history of relationships, about his early childhood—but everything was arranged, tidy, narratively complete. And yet, in one session, as he described a casual comment from a partner, he paused. "It's nothing," he said, "but it got under my skin." That phrase—"under my skin"—had never appeared before. It had texture. It suggested something unarranged.

When I invited him to linger there, he shrugged. "I don't want to go there," he said. Then, after a silence, "It's not even a real memory. I just... feel like I've been left before I ever arrived." He looked confused. It was neither a disclosure nor a breakthrough. It was a crack. What followed was not narrative but silence, then a reversion to the familiar curation. But something had shifted. The false self had trembled, not collapsed. It had let something through—not fully formed, not even symbolic, but *traced*. The fear of breakdown was not a future event. It was a structure in the room, a presence that could now be partially shared.

Galit Atlas, in her work on emotional inheritance, explores how secrecy lives not only in the individual but in the transgenerational field. The patient may carry affects, longings, and silences that are not strictly theirs. The false self often manages these inherited burdens—finding ways to keep symbolic space navigable when too much would otherwise leak through. For many queer patients, this includes legacies of shame, invisibility, or psychic splitting handed down not only through family but through culture.

This is where the false self and the closet intersect. As Eve Sedgwick taught us, the closet is not simply a space of concealment. It is a performative structure—one that manages visibility and erasure, speech and silence, being and non-being. The curated self, within this frame, is not hiding a truth. It is managing symbolic thresholds. It performs, yes—but in doing so, it keeps the self from breaking open. The closet is not the absence of experience. It is the container for **unformulated experience**—a psychic field shaped by what could not be metabolized in real time.

José Muñoz pushes this further, suggesting that performance is not a cover but a projection—an anticipatory structure. The self we perform may not exist yet, but we perform it in hopes that it will. The false self, then, becomes a site of possibility—a space where the unsymbolized might take shape. What is curated is not inauthentic. It is *not yet*.

The analyst's task is not to collapse this structure but to enter it with reverence. There is a deep ethical demand here—to recognize that what feels artificial may also be holding trauma, non-being, or memory without narrative. The patient may not need interpretation. They may need accompaniment. As Donna Orange writes, the analyst must become a witness—not to content alone, but to the conditions under which content becomes possible.

Winnicott helps us again. His idea that the feared breakdown is a trace of a non-experience allows us to recast symptoms not as distortions, but as communications from a part of the psyche that was never named. The false self, in this reading, is the keeper of these traces. It preserves affect without symbol. It manages the rhythm of disclosure, timing, pacing, and containment.

Bollas's concept of the *crypt* is useful here. In the absence of a receptive other, the psyche buries experience. Not repressed, not denied—buried. These crypts are curated by the false self, who keeps the psychic space organized, even if at a cost. When the analyst is too quick to "uncover" truth, they risk desecrating the symbolic logic of that burial. The goal is not excavation but **companioning**—to be with what has been hidden until it is ready to return.

The paradox is that secrecy can be deeply relational. The patient may test the analyst's willingness to remain outside the vault—to honor the sanctity of the hidden. When that respect is offered, sometimes the door opens. But it opens on its own time. It opens only when the holding is good enough.

This is not a call for therapeutic passivity. It is a call for precision, patience, and ethical attunement. The false self is not simply a defense against vulnerability. It is a **symbolic architecture built to house the unlivable**. And in time, it may become more porous—but only if it is respected. The fear of breakdown is real. It has already happened. And it will return again and again until the analyst is able to hold not the memory, but the absence. Not the story, but the trace.

Coda: The Ethics of Living Symbolically

The arc of this chapter has not aimed to resolve the split between the true and false self, but to inhabit it—to understand it as the very medium through which subjectivity unfolds. If there is something called authenticity, it does not lie in the eradication of the false self. It lives in the way we relate to our curated forms—the symbols, gestures, silences, and aesthetic arrangements we use to become recognizable to ourselves and others. It lives in our capacity to live symbolically.

To live symbolically is to surrender the fantasy of directness. It is to recognize that we are always mediated—by language, by history, by fantasy, by the internal presence of others. The false self is not a betrayal of this reality; it is one of its earliest expressions. When treated with respect, it can become less rigid, more poetic. Less a façade, more a frame. The analyst's task is not to dismantle it, but to enter its logic—to understand its syntax, to feel its rhythms, to listen to the story it is not quite telling.

The ethical demand here is subtle but profound. It asks us to abandon the wish for purity—to resist the temptation to distinguish too cleanly between what is false and what is true. Patients do not become real by being stripped bare. They become real when their curations are received with enough symbolic generosity that something unscripted can begin to appear. That appearance may be small—a hesitation, a different cadence, an unpracticed gesture. It is not a revelation, but a *reverberation*—the sound of something previously unvoiced echoing in a newly receptive space.

As therapists, we are asked to witness not only the content of the patient's life, but its form—the very architecture by which they have survived. When we respond to a patient's curated self with curiosity instead of frustration, something shifts. We become co-curators. We tend to the fragile exhibition together. We learn to read the performance not as avoidance, but as offering. And we begin to wonder: what is being kept safe here? What is being signaled in disguise?

The false self, in this light, is not inauthentic. It is *symbolic*. It shows what it cannot say. It performs as a way to preserve. And eventually, perhaps, it softens. Not because it is unmasked, but because it is no longer alone.

In the final sessions of treatment—or sometimes just in a fleeting moment that never quite recurs—a patient may say something not previously speakable. But it does not feel like a confession. It feels like music. A phrase, a silence, a glance that lands differently. The analyst does not respond with an interpretation. There is nothing to decode. Instead, we stay near. We accompany. We hold the space in which symbolic life has become more possible.

This is the ethical core of our work: not to strip away what has protected, but to join it. To recognize that the curated self was always a gesture—a longing for contact, carried in form. The real self, if it exists, does not arrive unmediated. It arrives in resonance.

Part 3

Recursive Integration and the Edge of Theory

10 The Original Paradox, Revisited

This chapter reflects on the psychoanalytic task of symbolizing the unlived—those dimensions of experience that were never metabolized, integrated, or spoken. It argues that the analyst's work is not to resolve paradox or heal fragmentation, but to remain present with what resists formulation. Drawing on Loewald, Bollas, Ogden, Winnicott, and Eigen, this chapter explores how psychic life exceeds ego structure and enters recursive, nonlinear forms. Psychoanalytic writing itself is reimagined as a holding environment, echoing the therapeutic posture of containment without closure. The analyst, like the writer, becomes a symbolic witness: one who listens to affect that has no narrative and helps it find form without forcing coherence. To symbolize the unlived is not to master it, but to love it into presence.

Recursive Openings: A Return Already in Motion

There are paradoxes that feel like wounds, and there are paradoxes that feel like birth. The original paradox—if there is such a thing—belongs to both. It recurs not as a question to be solved but as a rhythm that insists: the self cannot emerge without division, yet it cannot live divided.

This chapter returns, but not to the beginning. It spirals back to what was never linear: the tangled braid of knowing and being, of presence and defense, of the self as both witness and concealment. What was introduced in the first treatment of *The Original Paradox*—that we are formed in contradiction, that coherence is never total, that truth may only be tolerable in fragments—is not repeated here, but thickened.

Like the ouroboros, the mythic serpent consuming its own tail, this chapter enacts a recursive motion: not a circling for comfort, but a coiling that metabolizes its own material. The ouroboros is not only a symbol of eternity—it is a symbol of self-referential digestion, of subjectivity folding back upon itself in order to become. And yet, each turn around the spiral marks a new texture, a new ethical pressure.

To revisit paradox is not to return to where one was. It is to encounter the reconfigured shape of one's own prior knowing. What was once a defense

DOI: 10.4324/9781003715283-14

may now be a site of revelation. What was once unbearable may now be unhealable and yet shareable.

We begin, then, with this: the paradox of defense itself—not as a shield against reality, but as a recursive strategy of preservation that becomes the architecture of psychic life. In this return, myth and metapsychology weave together not as decoration, but as evidence.

Defense, in the psychoanalytic tradition, is often spoken of in terms of compromise: a negotiation between inner pressure and outer constraint, between impulse and adaptation. But what if defense is not a compromise, but a form of creation? What if it is not the symptom of failure, but the signature of survival?

Here, Freud's own mythological orientation becomes instructive. He turned to Oedipus not for the literal mechanics of family drama, but because the myth staged the unlivability of unknowing—how a truth too close to the self cannot be borne until it is catastrophically enacted. He reached for Narcissus to illuminate the implosion of subjectivity upon itself, the way in which the gaze turned inward becomes both mirror and grave.

We follow Freud, then, not in his conclusions but in his method: the search for psychic truths encoded in myth. If Oedipus and Narcissus were his symbolic companions, let ours be Cassandra, Dionysus, and the ouroboros.

Cassandra, cursed to speak true prophecies that no one would believe, is the mouthpiece of primary process thinking—fluid, associative, prophetic, and refused. Her tragedy is not only that she knows, but that her knowing cannot be metabolized by the symbolic order. Her speech, like the unconscious, is dismissed even as it haunts. She is the analyst's shadow figure: feelingful, predictive, accurate, and disbelieved.

Dionysus, god of ecstasy and dismemberment, offers a counterpoint. He is the embodiment of secondary process overrun—not as pure logic, but as integration gone wild. The rites of Dionysus do not suppress primary process—they stage it. Through wine, dance, and ecstatic rupture, Dionysian ritual fragments the body to reveal the divine in pieces. He is not the god of wholeness, but of revelation through collapse.

And then the ouroboros—neither god nor prophet, but the form of paradox itself. It devours to preserve, closes the circle to make it endless, and protects life by enacting its own threat. It is the perfect figure for what this chapter will explore: how defense both destroys and maintains and how subjectivity is not a fixed entity but a loop of becoming wrapped around its own impossibility.

Within this field, we begin to see that defense is not against danger—it is against the self's intensity. It is the organism's way of recoiling from its own aliveness, its own unformulated force.

The psyche, in this view, is not a container for reality, but a condensation of recursive gestures meant to manage its own unfolding. Defense is not a block to truth—it is truth in a condensed, coiled form. DNA, after all, is itself a paradox: the most expansive information held in the smallest spiral. A map of life twisted so tightly upon itself that it must be unwrapped to be expressed.

We are not selves. We are spirals of defense and disclosure, each act of becoming wrapped in a gesture of refusal. We grow not despite our paradoxes, but through them.

And what of epistemology and ontology? What of the difference between knowing and being, which psychoanalysis has long tried to keep clear? That, too, collapses here. In the paradoxical field, to know is already to be implicated. To feel is already to know something. The epistemic and the ontological are not sequential but entangled.

The patient does not first discover their truth and then become. They become through the process of partial discovery. And always in the presence of a witness who cannot extract without affecting, who cannot know without being known.

This section, then, opens the chapter not with a thesis, but with a mood: an atmosphere of recursive return, in which each concept will be re-entered, re-experienced, and recast. The next section will deepen this architecture of defense-as-creation, tracing how even our most primitive defenses preserve what they seem to destroy.

We will see that preservation is not about memory, but about form. That the split, the repression, the fragmentation—these are not erasures. They are inscriptions in a language that cannot yet be spoken, but must nevertheless be held.

And so we descend, again, not into chaos, but into complexity. The paradox is not the problem. It is the path.

Defenses That Preserve: The Architecture of Psychic Recoil

If we were to take seriously the idea that defense is not merely protective but creative, we would have to rethink the moral valence so often assigned to it. We speak casually of defenses as obstacles: primitive ones to be outgrown, mature ones to be strengthened. But what if this evolutionary framing misses something essential? What if every defense—no matter how splitting, bizarre, or regressive—also encodes the very psychic material it conceals?

This is not to romanticize pathology. It is to restore an aesthetic and ethical respect for the ingenuity of the psyche under threat. Even the most primitive defense is an act of psychic preservation. It does not annihilate the affect, it wards off—it reconfigures its terms of survival.

Repression does not erase the unbearable; it layers it into time. Projection does not discard danger; it places it into view at a distance. Dissociation does not destroy feeling; it freezes it into a symbolically encrypted trace. Each defense is a gesture of simultaneous refusal and retention. It destroys in order to preserve and preserves in order not to die.

In this light, defense becomes a kind of poetics. It is not a blunt instrument, but a structure of condensation. And in that condensation lives the germ of truth, twisted tightly around the very axis that denies it. The psyche recoils not only from danger, but from its own capacity to be overwhelmed by life.

This is where the paradox of psychic recoil emerges. The very force of vitality—libidinal, affective, primary-process intensity—threatens the fragile forms into which the self has been poured. And so the self, sensing this threat, recoils. But in recoiling, it preserves. Not the experience, but the potential for experience. Not memory, but trace.

We see this most clearly in defenses that appear destructive on their surface. Take splitting, for example. Often maligned as immature or pathological, splitting is not simply a failure to integrate. It is a way of preserving unbearable contradiction by holding it apart. The psyche cannot hold the mother as both loving and withholding, the analyst as both attuned and missed—and so it splits. But in doing so, it keeps both pieces alive. They are not yet capable of integration, but they have not been foreclosed. Splitting is not the absence of synthesis; it is the precondition for its future.

In the same way, denial is not an absence of knowing—it is a disavowed knowing. The flat refusal to acknowledge a loss, an illness, a betrayal often coexists with another part of the self that knows perfectly well. The paradox is maintained through a partition. This split is not a flaw; it is a sophisticated solution. It allows knowing and not-knowing to coexist in proximity, without collapse. Denial is a boundary drawn not between truth and falsehood, but between two truths that cannot yet coexist.

Even somatization, often regarded as a primitive defense, preserves through enactment what cannot be verbalized. The body becomes the parchment for an unformed symbol. The headache, the tightening gut, the skin flare—each is a script in a language the psyche does not yet know how to read. To say this is not to reduce the physical to the psychological, but to honor the body as a site of symbolic condensation. The symptom is not random; it is a monument to unspeakable experience.

If we look closely, we find that every defense participates in a paradoxical architecture of survival: it cuts to shield, splits to hold, silences to preserve. Defense does not merely shut down—it shapes. And what it shapes is often the form of the subject itself.

Here we might return to Freud, but not to his metapsychology of drives alone. Rather, to his aesthetic sensibility—the way he viewed the symptom as a compromise-formation, a layered expression of clashing forces that nevertheless speaks. In *The Interpretation of Dreams*, Freud emphasizes that the dream-work disguises wish and conflict not to obliterate them, but to render them tolerable to consciousness. The disguise is not betrayal; it is craft. The same applies to defense: it allows what would otherwise shatter the psyche to arrive in symbolic form.

Klein, too, intuited this. In her work on the paranoid-schizoid and depressive positions, the movement from splitting and projection toward integration is not framed as a linear advancement but as an oscillation. Even in adulthood, the psyche returns to primitive positions. And not because it is weak, but because certain realities are perpetually hard to bear. The child—and later, the adult—preserves love through hate, presence through absence, connection through rupture. The defense is not a betrayal of the object, but a desperate means of staying in relation to it.

And what of mature defenses? Sublimation, humor, and anticipation—often praised for their adaptability—are not immune to paradox. In sublimation, the unacceptable drive is transformed into a socially permitted expression. But the transformation retains the drive's intensity. The artwork, the philosophical argument, the clinical insight—each bears the imprint of what was once unbearable. The form is changed, but the heat remains. The drive survives through symbolic expression. Defense becomes expression.

Even humor, which appears to release tension, does not dispel it. It reframes it. A joke allows the unspeakable to emerge through a linguistic side door. It permits contact with affect without being overwhelmed. Laughter is not only release—it is the sound of the unbearable made briefly survivable.

What binds these disparate defenses together is their formal structure: they all recoil in order to preserve. Like the ouroboros, they turn inward—not to collapse, but to continue. Their preservation is not static; it is dynamic, spiraling, recursive.

In clinical work, this understanding shifts our posture. We do not aim to strip away defenses, as though they were obstructions to truth. We learn to read them as inscriptions—marks left by the self on the wall of survival. To interpret a defense is not to puncture it, but to trace its contours with reverence. The goal is not exposure, but gradual dilation: the widening of space within which contradiction can breathe.

And here, too, the analyst must resist a certain idealization of coherence. Integration is not always the task. Sometimes the work is to hold the fragments without fusing them. To let denial remain a little longer, to respect the timing of the psyche's unfolding. As Eigen reminds us, there are truths that require patience to be born. The analyst waits, not for the right interpretation, but for the moment when the psyche begins to feel safe enough to loosen its coil.

We might think of defense, then, as a kind of internal choreography—movements learned under duress, repeated with such frequency that they become identity. To undo them too quickly is to unravel the very form that makes experience tolerable. The task is not to dismantle the dance, but to hear its music, to sense when it might shift.

This is the architecture of psychic recoil. It does not stand in the way of the self—it is the self, in the moment before it can arrive.

What comes next is a deepening of this coil: a reflection on the symbolizing process itself. How does the self emerge not just through defense, but through symbolic wrapping—a condensation of intensity, like DNA, folded into forms that preserve it even while they obscure it?

We turn now to the subject as a symbol of itself—not as a metaphor, but as a paradoxical condition.

"We Are All Symbols of Ourselves": Condensation, Selfhood, and the Fold

To speak of the self as a symbol is to acknowledge that what we experience as identity is never fully present. It is deferred, wrapped, and condensed. Like a text that can only be read in translation, the self arrives already encoded—shaped by history, culture, family, memory, and defense. We are not what we are. We are how we survive being what we are.

In Freud's dream theory, condensation is a primary mechanism by which the unconscious expresses itself. Multiple latent thoughts are compressed into a single manifest image. One figure in a dream may carry traces of several people, conflicts, wishes—folded into each other, their distinctness blurred but not erased. The dream does not lie; it abbreviates. It symbolically compresses truths that cannot be spoken directly.

What if the self functions similarly? Not as a singular coherence, but as a condensation of multiple psychic vectors—some known, some unknown, some long ago exiled. What we call "I" is not a stable referent but a compressed symbol: a Möbius strip of memory and defense, desire and containment, wound and compensation. This is not pathology, it is structure.

And this structure is protective. Just as DNA coils itself into the tight helix of chromatin to preserve and regulate its expression, the self folds its psychic material to remain intact. Trauma, longing, shame, aggression, joy—each is tucked into symbol, into symptom, into character. The very shape of our subjectivity is an architecture of containment.

From this angle, every presentation of self is a kind of glyph: an encrypted form that both reveals and conceals. Even speech—our most direct medium of expression—functions symbolically. It does not transmit the self; it gestures toward it. The analyst, like the dream interpreter, listens not for content alone, but for condensation—for the affect that leaks through syntax, for the unspoken that pulses beneath the said.

We are, in this sense, always folded. Not only in the aftermath of trauma, but by virtue of subjectivity itself. Our existence is recursive. We reflect on our thoughts, narrate our feelings, name our desires—always a step removed from the immediacy of experience. To be a subject is to be split.

Derrida's *différance* speaks to this: the meaning of a word, or a self, is never fully present in the moment. It is always postponed, always deferred, dependent on a chain of other signs for its intelligibility. The self, too, is a deferral—a placeholder for a coherence that never fully arrives.

This is not a loss. It is a richness. The folded self is not an illusion to be undone, but a form to be honored. It holds contradiction without collapse. It allows multiple versions of the self to coexist—not as fragments, but as echoes within a single symbolic form.

And yet, we often treat this folding as failure. We speak of "authenticity," "integration," "cohesion" as ideals—as if the true self were a singular, unmediated presence. But what if the most authentic self is the one that remains layered? Not disorganized, but multiply organized. Not incoherent, but polyphonic.

The analyst, too, is folded. In the transference field, they are witness, participant, symbol, object, ghost. Their subjectivity is not bracketed—it is shaped, invoked, condensed. To speak in the analytic setting is to speak from within a mutual coil: each voice inflected by histories that are not fully known, by affects that cannot be located, by meanings that emerge only in relation.

To work psychoanalytically is to attend to this layering—not to peel it back in search of some unvarnished core, but to feel its texture. To listen not only to what is said, but to what folds within the saying. The patient who jokes in a moment of grief, who intellectualizes in a moment of shame, is not avoiding. They are folding affect into symbol—making it survivable.

Michael Eigen calls this the density of aliveness: the psychic substance that accrues when we allow contradiction to persist without resolution. For Eigen, the self is not an entity, but a field—pulsing, pressured, reverberating. A field that holds its own unknowability as part of its depth.

This unknowability is not an absence. It is a protection. To know the self too fully is, perhaps, to fix it—to collapse the wave of possibility into a particle of certainty. And so we remain, necessarily, symbols of ourselves. Not because we are hiding, but because we are complex.

The myth of Narcissus offers a cautionary echo. He sees his reflection and takes it for substance. He falls in love not with another, but with the appearance of self. But the mirror does not speak. It does not return gaze with gaze. He cannot fold into it; he can only drown.

The analytic mirror must be different. It must not flatten the patient into reflection. It must hold their foldedness and allow their condensation to speak. The analyst does not reflect back a self-image; they reverberate with it. They become a second symbolizer—someone who helps preserve the form without collapsing it into definition.

We might think here, too, of the ouroboros—the snake that eats its own tail, the symbol of recursive eternity. It is often taken as a sign of unity, but unity through folding. It contains itself by devouring itself and preserves itself through self-erasure. This is the paradox of symbolization: we construct ourselves by looping back on what we once were, what we might be, what we never were at all.

The self as ouroboros is not self-consuming in a destructive sense, but self-enfolding. A topology of becoming that has no outside. It holds itself in recursion, not in order to disappear, but to remain alive.

In the analytic process, we attend to these folds not to unfold them entirely, but to thicken their meaning. We listen for condensation, not to unpack it into clarity, but to accompany its density. We come to feel that every moment of psychic life is symbolic—not in a metaphorical sense, but structurally. Even silence is symbolic. Even a symptom. Even the unsaid.

And so we arrive at a paradox: to be real is to be symbolic. To be oneself is to be a translation of oneself. We are not falsifying experience by folding it—we are preserving it. Like DNA, our psychic material is coiled not for hiding, but for continuity. Wrapped to endure.

To love someone, in this light, is to love their folding. Not their nakedness alone, but their complexity. To allow their condensation to remain partially encrypted. To read the text of them without demanding that it be glossed.

The analyst, then, is not a decoder. They are a reader of symbols. A keeper of folds. A companion to the condensed self.

We are all symbols of ourselves. And psychoanalysis, at its most reverent, learns not to unfold us too quickly.

Myth as Recursive Topology: Ouroboros, Dionysus, Cassandra

If the psyche folds upon itself to preserve aliveness, then myth may be its oldest map—an encoded topology of paradox. Myths do not teach; they reverberate. They hold contradiction without resolving it, staging psychic impasses in symbolic form. Freud turned to Oedipus and Narcissus not because they offered clear origin stories, but because they condensed something unlivable into a narrative container. What myth offers is not meaning, but mood—an affective architecture for experiences that resist integration. In this sense, myth is not explanatory. It is recursive. It returns where thought breaks down.

Among the most potent of these recursive myths is the Ouroboros, the ancient symbol of the snake devouring its own tail. It is not a circle, but a paradox: life sustained through self-consumption, continuity through return. The Ouroboros is not about wholeness in the classical sense. It is about folded persistence—a form that survives not in spite of recursion, but through it.

The psychic life of many patients echoes this loop. They repeat symptoms not because they have failed to move forward, but because forward motion was foreclosed. They turn back upon themselves in fantasy, in addiction, in rage—not as regression, but as preservation. Their defenses are not misguided—they are recursive solutions to unbearable contradiction. In such cases, analysis does not untangle the loop. It slows it, witnesses it, and makes space for a symbol to emerge within it.

The Ouroboros is also a topology of defense. It conceals what it contains. The snake swallows itself not to end, but to keep what is inner from becoming outer. This is the logic of dissociation, of psychic enclosure. The self protects itself from its own intensity by looping inwards, preserving energy in symbolic suspension. A patient who cannot cry in the presence of the analyst but weeps in dreams, or in fantasy, is not resisting—they are folded. Their affect lives in a loop they dare not interrupt.

This is why defenses are not simply barriers. They are also cradles. They destroy while preserving. They disavow affect in order to protect the self from psychic combustion. But they do not erase the affect. They loop it, compress it, and symbolically suspend it. What we call pathology may be the psyche's most enduring topology: the recursive preservation of what could not be metabolized.

Dionysus, god of ecstasy and madness, offers a second topology. If the Ouroboros symbolizes recursive preservation, Dionysus embodies ecstatic rupture. Born from a violent dismembering—twice-born, from mother and father—he arrives not as synthesis, but as contradiction incarnate: the god of intoxication, of boundary-loss, of divine madness. In the psychoanalytic imagination, Dionysus is the force of primary process: irrational, fluid, timeless. He does not narrate—he overwhelms.

But Dionysus is not pure chaos. He is also disguised. His madness is staged, ritualized. The Dionysian rites were forms of symbolic re-entry—spaces in which the self could dissolve, but not be annihilated. This is the paradox of regression in analysis: to lose coherence not as failure, but as symbolic return. Dionysian states are not departures from the self; they are enactments of what the self had to abandon.

In analytic work, patients may enter Dionysian states without knowing it: a sudden tearfulness, a fragment of fantasy, a lapse in speech that floods with emotion. These are not regressions to be corrected. They are ritual moments, temporary suspensions of the defended self, in which affect can arrive out of sequence. Dionysus does not heal; he breaks open. But his breaking is in the service of feeling. He is not the analyst—but he is what the analyst must sometimes tolerate in the room.

The third figure is Cassandra, the cursed prophetess of Troy. Given the gift of foresight, she is doomed never to be believed. She knows, but cannot persuade. She speaks the truth, but her speech is structurally unhearable. Cassandra is the myth of unintegrated knowing—primary process trapped in a secondary process world. She does not symbolize affect; she channels it. And her audience, like the analyst, too early or too defensively, misses the meaning because it arrives in a form they cannot bear.

Cassandra is the myth of the patient who knows too much, too early. Who intuits, senses, prophesies—who tells of betrayal before it is visible, of danger before it is clear. However, when this knowledge is not met with containment, it becomes a curse. They are dismissed as dramatic, as hysterical, as untrustworthy. Their speech, though saturated with truth, is unreceived.

In clinical work, Cassandra appears as the patient whose insight is uncannily accurate—but unfelt. They narrate trauma, betrayal, and self-abandonment with precision, but without affect. Their knowledge is not integrated—it is foreclosed truth, spoken from exile. The analyst may be tempted to admire their intellect or match it. But what Cassandra needs is not agreement. She needs accompaniment—someone to hear what has long been heard only by herself.

We are all, in some ways, Ouroboros, Dionysus, and Cassandra. We fold into ourselves to survive, we dissolve to feel, we speak what cannot be heard. These myths are not simply stories; they are psychic structures. The analyst's task is not to decode them, but to recognize them when they recur—in gesture, in silence, in dream, in defense.

To think mythopoetically in analysis is to grant depth to the symbolic life of the patient—not as metaphor, but as method. Myth provides a topology of the unspeakable. It stages psychic truths in forms the psyche can bear. The child who dissociates to survive may one day dream of a snake eating its tail. The adult who rages without cause may be caught in Dionysian ecstasy, seeking a feeling they never had permission to name. The patient who narrates their pain without affect may be speaking from the mouth of Cassandra.

And so we do not interpret the myth away. We listen to it. We allow it to shape our sense of the field. When a patient offers a symbol, an image, or a dream, we do not ask, "What does it mean?" We ask: "How is it living in the room now?"

Myths are not the past. They are the recursive forms the psyche adopts to remain alive under pressure. They encode contradiction, protect affect, and offer a symbolic space for the unlivable to be staged. The Ouroboros contains, Dionysus dissolves, and Cassandra cries out. Each holds a facet of the analytic encounter.

If we are to write a psychoanalysis attuned to paradox, we must allow these mythic forms to guide us—not as doctrine, but as atmosphere. They remind us that the psyche is not linear. It loops. It bursts. It mourns in advance. It prophesies without being heard. It turns back in order to go forward. And it often survives by symbolizing what it could not yet feel.

The mythic is not an escape from reality. It is a condensed truth—a psychic short form for the long arc of becoming.

Against Integration: The Ethics of Nonclosure

Psychoanalysis has long privileged integration. To bring the unconscious into consciousness, to convert passive into active, to make what was split whole—these have been guiding imperatives. But what if wholeness is not always the aim? What if some forms of psychic truth can only survive by remaining unintegrated?

To argue against integration is not to valorize fragmentation. It is to ask whether integration, when overvalued, becomes a subtler form of domination—a secondary process ideal imposed on psychic life that may, paradoxically, erase the very complexity it seeks to hold. This chapter proposes that nonclosure—what cannot be reconciled, metabolized, or fully symbolized—is not a failure of therapy, but a form of ethical fidelity to the patient's psychic structure. Especially when that structure is built, as in so many of the chapters in this book, upon paradox.

We return here to the idea of defense. In traditional metapsychology, defense serves to protect the ego from overwhelming instinctual conflict. But there are deeper readings. Defense, in its most primordial form, protects the self from the self—from the unlivable reality of its own intensity. It is not a wall against the world. It is a coil around an unthinkable core.

To defend is to preserve something unbearable, not destroy it. It is a loop, not a cut. The psyche bends, recedes, fragments—not to expel reality, but to survive it. As such, defense contains an ethic of its own. It is an act of inner conservation. Even in its most pathological form, it keeps something safe in suspension. To dissolve it too quickly in the name of coherence is to miss the logic of its formation.

This understanding reorients the analyst's task. We are not surgeons removing pathological structures. We are witnesses to the architecture of preservation. In this light, the aim of analysis is not integration, but symbolization. Not unity, but a survivable form.

Many patients live in states that defy integration. Dissociative states, recursive shame, affective foreclosure—these are not fragments waiting to be stitched together. They are alternate forms of cohesion, provisional architectures of survival. The patient who performs in session, then dissociates in private, is not "resisting." They are maintaining a split that has allowed their subjectivity to endure.

To ask such a patient to integrate too quickly—to bring all parts into dialogue, to collapse contradiction into narrative—can feel like violence. It risks annihilating the affective realities that those parts were created to contain. Loewald understood this when he wrote of the "depth dimension" of time in psychoanalysis. What appears as incoherence in the present may, over time, reveal a deeper psychic order—not through explanation, but through patient dwelling.

There is an ontological humility here. To be a psychoanalyst is not to know, but to remain with what is not yet knowable. The analyst becomes, in Ogden's terms, a participant-observer of psychic life, not its master. We accompany the self not into unity, but into greater complexity. And we learn to listen for the places where integration would constitute a form of betrayal.

This is especially true in work with patients who organize around foreclosure. Their psychic reality is not organized around lack, but around absence—what was never there, never symbolized, never allowed to arrive. For such patients, the task is not to retrieve what was lost, but to symbolically witness what never had form. To do this is to resist the analyst's own impulse toward narrative closure. It is to accept that some truths must remain partial, suspended, glimpsed only through affective resonance.

This is not pessimism. It is a different arc of therapeutic possibility. Freud himself was ambivalent about cure. In his late work, he suggested that analysis was successful not when it produced insight, but when it allowed patients to transform misery into common unhappiness. A modest goal, but perhaps also a radical one. To live alongside one's paradoxes, without collapsing them, may be the truest form of change.

Nonclosure also protects the erotic dimension of analytic work. The erotic is not simply sexual—it is the field of desire, of movement, of unfulfilled longing. To integrate the erotic too completely is to risk domesticating it. But to allow it to remain partially unresolved—to let it pulse, reverberate, shift—preserves its generativity. The erotic does not seek resolution. It seeks recognition.

This stance echoes Jessica Benjamin's vision of mutual recognition—not fusion, not separation, but the dynamic play between self and other. The goal is not to become one, but to remain two—held in a field of tension that is alive, unfinished. In analytic terms, this means that the analyst does not rush to interpret, but holds open the space in which the patient's multiple self-states can begin to coexist.

This ethic also reverberates in post-structuralist thought. Derrida's *différance*, for instance, reminds us that meaning is always deferred, never complete. To "know" the self is always a retroactive act, filtered through language, shaped by absence. Likewise, Foucault cautioned that the self is not a thing to be discovered, but a site of inscription—a product of power, discourse, and resistance. Integration, from this view, is not liberation—it may be assimilation.

To write—and practice—with this in mind is to honor the fragments. It is to stay close to the patient's psychic idiom, even when it resists formulation. It is to respect the timeline of symbolic life, which rarely moves in straight lines. It is to understand that the patient who pauses before naming a feeling may not be resisting—they may be protecting its nascent form.

We return, then, to the opening paradox of this book: that some psychic truths must remain unstable in order to be real. That to stabilize them prematurely is to falsify their texture. That paradox is not an error, but a topology of becoming.

To live without full integration is not to be broken. It is to live in time, in rhythm, in recursive tension with what one cannot fully absorb. This is not a deficit. It is a form of attunement. And the analyst's ethical task is to hold space for that attunement—not to fix it, but to love it into form.

The Subject as Symbol: Condensation, Recoil, and the Self as Artifact

In the analytic encounter, we often speak of the "self" as though it were a coherent entity, a protagonist with inner depth, narrative continuity, and integrative potential. But the self, when followed closely, begins to dissolve into symbol—an artifact of relational encounter, a residue of internalized gaze, a structure shaped as much by absence as by presence. This section proposes that subjectivity is not a fixed interiority but a symbolic artifact: coiled, condensed, recoiled upon itself, often wrapped protectively to survive its own intensity.

We are not selves. We are renderings—provisional images through which we make ourselves intelligible to others and to ourselves. In this sense, we are all, to some degree, symbols of ourselves. And like any symbol, the self is both expressive and elusive: it communicates something essential while obscuring what cannot yet be said. This dual function—of revealing and protecting—lies at the heart of psychic survival.

Freud knew this when he turned to myth. Oedipus and Narcissus were not just clinical metaphors; they were condensations of structural truth. Oedipus, in uncovering the truth of his desire, blinds himself. Knowledge cannot be borne in the register of sight. Narcissus, in trying to love himself, finds only a surface that cannot return the gaze. He perishes not from self-love, but from the impossibility of being held by his own reflection. Both myths encode the paradox of subjectivity: to know oneself is to risk destruction; to seek oneself is to encounter a representation.

In this spirit, we turn to a different set of myths: the Ouroboros, Dionysus, and Cassandra. Each reveals something elemental about the symbolic self—the ways it coils to protect its core, splits under excess, or speaks truths no one is willing to hear.

The **Ouroboros**, the serpent devouring its own tail, is perhaps the most enduring image of recursive psychic life. It is not only a symbol of eternity—it is a map of psychic defense. The subject turns back upon itself not to annihilate, but to contain. This self-consuming motion mirrors the function of certain defenses: projection that doubles back as identification, repression that returns as symptom, dissociation that becomes structure. The Ouroboric self is neither linear nor fragmented. It is circular, recursive, looping through past and present without resolution.

In clinical work, this often appears as compulsive re-enactment—patients who loop through the same dynamics, not because they resist insight, but because the motion itself is preserving something unrepresentable. The repetition is not regression. It is symbolic protection. The self devours its tail to keep itself from dissolving.

Dionysus, by contrast, represents psychic excess. He is not symbolic containment, but symbolic shattering. The god of wine, ecstasy, and madness—Dionysus incarnates the parts of the psyche that cannot be tamed by reason. In myth, he is born twice: once from the womb of Semele, and once from the thigh of Zeus, after his body has been torn apart. His followers engage in ritual madness, his rites transgress social order, and his presence destabilizes identity. He is not integrated—he is possessed.

Dionysus shows us what happens when secondary process collapses under the pressure of primary process, when affect surges without a container. When the symbolic order gives way to the rawness of affective intensity, and yet he is not simply chaos. He is reborn through rupture. He is the part of thc psyche that resists being pinned down, that refuses closure, that demands symbolic recognition even in its most disorganized form.

To work analytically in Dionysian territory is to tolerate breakdown—not as failure, but as emergence. It is to remain present with patients in states of disintegration, psychotic anxiety, ecstatic dissociation—not in order to quickly restore order, but to listen for what is being born in the wreckage. Dionysus does not bring integration. He brings the possibility of symbolic reassembly after dismemberment.

Cassandra, the cursed prophetess of Greek myth, was given the power to see the future but was cursed never to be believed. She speaks the truth, but her truth is inadmissible to the symbolic order. In psychoanalytic terms, she represents the aspect of the psyche that knows too early, too deeply, too truly—but cannot be heard. She is the voice of the primary process operating in a world governed by secondary process constraints. Her speech is affective, nonlinear, disturbing—and thus disavowed.

Cassandra haunts the analytic setting. The patient who names the truth of their experience but feels invalidated. The analyst who senses something in the transference but doubts its admissibility. The prophetic utterance in a dream or slip of the tongue that reveals more than the ego can hold. In each, we see the tension between psychic truth and symbolic legibility. Cassandra's tragedy is not that she is mad, but that the world cannot tolerate her form of knowing.

This points us toward a deeper paradox: epistemology and ontology are not separate. Knowing and being are co-constituted. The way we are permitted to know ourselves shapes how we are allowed to be. And when certain forms of knowing—feeling, affective resonance, bodily truth—are denied symbolic registration, our being becomes structured around absence. The self becomes a condensation of disavowed knowing—a symbol of a symbol, folded in defense.

This brings us back to defense as a mode of symbolic architecture. Defense is not simply repression. It is a form of psychic design—protecting the unbearable not by destroying it, but by encoding it in symbolic form. A symptom, a gesture, a posture, a silence—all may function as encrypted truths. These are not communication failures. They are aesthetic compressions, ways the psyche condenses intensity into survivable shapes.

Like **DNA**, the self coils—not to obscure, but to conserve. The double helix is not chaos. It is density. A code so densely wound that it carries the blueprint of life in microscopic form. So too with the symbolic self: what appears as muteness may be saturation; what looks like blankness may be condensation. To unfold such structures requires not interpretation, but presence. Not clarity, but reverence.

To think of the subject as a symbol is to relinquish the fantasy of full access. We do not find the "real self" beneath the defenses. We find a structure of folds—each layer protecting, revealing, transforming the one beneath. The analyst does not uncover. They accompany the unfolding. They sit with the symbols long enough for them to become animate.

In this view, analytic work is not the restoration of a core self, but the recognition of a symbolic self—crafted under pressure, shaped by absence, held together by condensation and recoil. The analyst becomes not an excavator, but a reader of artifacts. A curator of fragments. A participant in the symbolic life of a self that is never fully present, but always arriving.

We are not selves. We are forms. We are recursions. We are the Ouroboros devouring its tail to preserve itself. We are the Dionysian fragment dancing at the edge of language. We are Cassandra, knowing without being known. And in the analytic field, we find the space not to resolve these images, but to let them breathe.

To see the subject as a symbol is to accept that psychic life does not need to make sense in order to matter. That meaning is not always integration, and that healing may involve living more fully into one's own symbolic architecture. The goal is not to make the self whole. It is to let the self remain strange—and to be met there.

The Analyst as Artifact: Presence, Rupture, and Symbolic Co-Construction

If the subject is a symbolic artifact—condensed, recursive, and shaped by disavowed intensities—then so too must the analyst be understood not as an observer outside the system, but as a figure within it. In this section, I propose that the analyst is not simply a witness to the patient's symbolic structure, but becomes part of it. The analyst is not only a container, but a symbolic surface onto which the patient's paradoxes are projected, enacted, and metabolized. In this way, the analyst becomes an artifact—created, discovered, and altered within the field of analytic encounter.

This reframes presence not as neutrality or technique, but as symbolic participation. The analyst's body, voice, timing, silences, and interpretive choices all become part of the patient's symbolic architecture. We are not simply working on the psyche; we are entering the psyche's aesthetic grammar. And if the self is always in some sense symbolic—coiled against itself, folded into representation—then the analyst is not an external observer but a recursive figure within that system.

The Analyst as Representational Surface

From the patient's vantage, the analyst is not a person but a surface—a reflective screen onto which affective intensities are cast. This is not transference in the classical sense, where past objects are replayed in the present. It is more radical: the analyst becomes the medium through which dissociated self-states are given temporary coherence. The analyst is not only the recipient of projection, but its expressive material. Our presence gives shape to what could not otherwise appear.

Consider a patient who enters the session with wordlessness, offering no material. The analyst waits. The silence lengthens. Finally, the patient says, "You're not saying anything because you think I'm too much." This moment is not simply a projection—it is a symbolic act. The analyst's silence has become a surface upon which the patient's feared excess is made visible. The analyst, in being experienced as critical, has become a symbol of containment's failure. But this symbol is not false. It is a live element in the patient's emotional ecology. The analyst must now inhabit the role—not to confirm it, but to hold its symbolic meaning long enough for it to be metabolized.

Symbolic Co-Creation and Rupture

When the analyst becomes an artifact of the patient's symbolic structure, the encounter becomes one of co-construction rather than interpretation. We do not uncover meaning—we participate in its formation. And this formation often involves rupture.

The analyst's misattunements, silences, or interventions may produce symbolic fractures—not because they are errors, but because they reveal the edge of the patient's symbolic tolerance. These ruptures are not mistakes to be repaired; they are events to be symbolized. They offer an opening into the architecture of the self—its limits, its thresholds, its defended contours.

In this way, the analytic field becomes a recursive structure: the patient constructs the analyst as a symbol, and the analyst, in being so constructed, offers the patient a new possibility of self-symbolization. It is not about being correct. It is about being symbolically available. What matters is not the analyst's intention, but their willingness to become part of the patient's recursive architecture—and to stay there long enough for something new to emerge.

The Analyst's Symbolic Unknowing

To enter this field requires a particular kind of humility. The analyst does not know who they are within the patient's symbolic world. We do not control the meanings projected onto us. We become teachers, lovers, ghosts, judges, and absences. These symbolic identities are not delusions. They are expressions of psychic truth.

Eigen writes of the analyst as a "tone of soul"—a presence that vibrates within the patient's emotional world. This tone is not factual; it is poetic. It registers not what we do, but what we mean in the symbolic economy of the patient's psyche. To work in this register requires not knowledge, but attunement. We do not need to know what we are; we need to feel what we are becoming.

Defense as Symbolic Gesture

Earlier, we explored defense as symbolic condensation. Here, we extend that logic: the analyst often becomes the object of those defenses—not because the patient wishes to push us away, but because their very structure requires it. The analyst becomes dangerous, alluring, empty, too much. These are not resistances to analysis. They are the analysis. They are symbolic gestures—enactments of what has never been spoken.

A patient once told me: "I want you to be close, but I need you to be far away." This contradiction was not a conflict to be resolved—it was a symbolic truth. I was not being asked to choose between presence and absence. I was being asked to inhabit the paradox. To become a symbol of the patient's unformulated yearning—a figure close enough to evoke, distant enough to survive.

The analyst, in this frame, is a symbolic construct coiled around the patient's need. We are not fixed objects. We are recursive mirrors, surfaces that reflect without collapse, containers that can be filled without dissolving. This is not to say we are blank screens. On the contrary, our subjectivity is precisely what allows us to be symbolized. We bring tone, rhythm, fragility, and timing. But these qualities do not make us opaque—they make us metabolizable.

The Ethics of Symbolic Participation

To become an artifact in the patient's symbolic system is not an invitation to surrender our clinical judgment. It is an ethical task. We must remain present enough to hold the symbolic projection without being overtaken by it. This requires restraint, clarity, and a willingness to acknowledge and tolerate our own distortions.

Loewald's concept of the "re-animation of psychic life" speaks to this process. The analyst does not animate the patient by injecting meaning into them. We animate the patient by becoming symbolically available—by offering a presence that can hold condensation, echo recursive movement, and tolerate recoil. We allow the patient to experience themselves not as a fixed self, but as a becoming. And in that becoming, the analyst becomes too.

Analyst as Symbolic Object in the Recursive Field

In the most transformative moments of analytic work, the analyst is not simply present. They are *used*—not as objects of need, but as symbolic elements in the patient's recursive field. This is the Winnicottian use of the object, reimagined. The patient destroys the analyst not in aggression, but in symbolization. They overwrite our presence with meaning. And if we survive this—if we remain symbolically intact despite the distortion—then something shifts. The patient experiences, perhaps for the first time, a self capable of representing affect rather than being undone by it.

To be an artifact is not to be passive. It is to be stable enough to hold paradox, porous enough to invite projection, and affectively attuned enough to metabolize symbolic experience. The analyst becomes a figure through which the patient rehearses not only past relationships but future possibilities of selfhood. We are a rehearsal space for becoming.

Recursive Time and the Ethics of Paradox

If the self is not a linear development but a recursive unfolding—if it is constituted through symbolic condensation, deferred metabolization, and representational recoil—then temporality itself must be rethought. Psychic life does not move forward through integration; it loops, fractures, and returns. The analyst does not work on a timeline of restoration, but inside a field where past, present, and future are co-constructed in nonlinear synchrony. In this section, we turn to time—not as sequence, but as a medium of paradox—and to the ethical stance required to work within it.

The Temporal Structure of the Symptom

Symptoms are not simply the return of the repressed. They are condensations of multiple temporalities: affect unprocessed, desire foreclosed, fragments of a past that was never fully lived. In this view, symptoms are *time-knots*—psychic events that carry traces of what has not yet happened, what happened too early, and what could not happen then but might yet happen now.

A patient describes a fantasy of being cradled like a baby, despite having no conscious memory of neglect. The fantasy carries with it grief, shame, and a wish so strong it becomes unbearable. In analysis, the fantasy does not point backward to an event; it opens a field of recursive time in which that event might still occur—not as a factual restoration, but as a symbolic arrival. The fantasy is not a regressive escape; it is a temporal demand.

Eigen speaks of trauma as "time breaking apart"—an experience that cannot be registered in sequence and thus persists as an ever-present absence. The analyst's role is not to return the patient to a timeline but to tolerate the brokenness of time, to become a presence within which recursive temporalities may resonate, collide, and refract.

Recursive Temporality and Symbolic Incompletion

This looping of time is not failure; it is structure. Just as the Ouroboros devours its tail not to end itself but to sustain its continuity, the psyche returns to its own fragments in order to hold itself together. Recursive temporality allows for psychic survival when forward motion would annihilate.

The Ouroboros, an ancient symbol found in Egyptian, Greek, and Hindu iconography, represents self-containment, repetition, and cyclical transformation. In our analytic context, it becomes the emblem of the patient who repeats not to remember, but to remain intact. Their psychic return is not pathological—it is ontological. They are structured by return. The analyst does not interpret this return as resistance, but as a gesture of paradoxical continuity: a re-engagement with what was never permitted to unfold.

This perspective reframes working through. Loewald described analytic time as deep time—not a forward progression but a temporal layering in which past and present interpenetrate. The symptom is not excavated; it is symbolically re-inscribed. The analyst holds a space not for resolution, but for recursive duration.

Dionysus and the Ethics of Fragmentation

To remain in recursive time is to accept that wholeness may not be the aim. Dionysus, the Greek god of ecstasy, dismemberment, and rebirth, embodies this principle. He is torn apart and reassembled, not as a return to prior integrity, but as a new form of subjectivity born of fragmentation. His myth encodes a symbolic truth: that integration is not always restorative; sometimes it is distorting. True psychic life may begin only after dismemberment.

For the patient, this means that healing may not feel cohesive. It may feel like aesthetic scatter, like emotional chaos. The analyst must bear this Dionysian intensity—not by ordering it, but by staying present to it. This is the ethics of analytic presence: to hold not only the parts that cohere, but those that rupture the field.

Here we must remember that psychoanalysis is not a technology of repair. It is an ethics of presence. The analyst must not rescue the patient from fragmentation too quickly, lest we foreclose the very experience that allows for symbolic life to re-emerge. Dionysus teaches us that psychic dismemberment is not the end; it is often the precondition for symbolic depth.

Cassandra and the Tragedy of Knowing without Being Heard

Where Dionysus embodies the ecstatic rupture of form, Cassandra—cursed to utter true prophecies that no one believes—embodies the tragedy of unrecognized knowledge. Her myth is a representation of what it means to carry knowing that cannot be metabolized by the other. She speaks in primary process; the culture hears in secondary process and rejects her.

Cassandra figures the analytic patient who speaks affectively, symbolically, dissociatively—but whose truth is too raw, too early, too outside the syntax of normative discourse. Her curse is not madness; it is misrecognition.

In analytic practice, Cassandra moments arise when the patient offers psychic truths that feel unbearable or incoherent—truths that the analyst may be tempted to soften, translate, or interpret prematurely. The ethical task is to let the Cassandra state exist without collapsing it into meaning. To hold knowing that cannot yet be heard. To witness without assimilating.

This is where the analyst must resist both mastery and rescue. We become, instead, the one who stays—who allows unhearable truths to reverberate until they find symbolic traction. Not all speech seeks understanding; some seeks company.

Epistemology and Ontology as Intertwined

All of this returns us to a central paradox: knowing and being are not separate. In analytic work, what is known is often what has not yet been lived, and what is lived often exceeds what can be known. To split epistemology and ontology—as Descartes might have done—is to miss the recursive loop between them.

Post-Heideggerian thought, especially in the work of Merleau-Ponty, shows us that being is always already perceptual, always entwined with the structures of how we make sense. In analysis, this becomes clear: the patient comes to know themselves through the experience of being with the analyst. The knowledge is not reflective; it is participatory. The self is constituted in the field.

To know something in analysis is not to master it cognitively. It is to become able to feel it in the presence of another. This is recursive knowing—not a linear accumulation of facts, but a spiraling into affective coherence. The analyst becomes a co-constitutor of this knowing-being field. We are not outside of it. We are of it.

The Ethics of Staying in Time

To work within recursive time is to forgo completion. The analyst does not offer final interpretations, linear trajectories, or cohesive identities. We offer a duration. We stay. We become the site at which fragments can return without being pathologized. We delay the collapse into coherence so that something more truthful might emerge.

This demands what Loewald called "temporal depth"—the capacity to hold not only the patient's story, but the patient's non-narrative experience. To recognize that what returns is not simply memory, but a temporal field seeking form. Our presence must not force this form. It must accompany it.

The analyst becomes, then, not a guide but a timekeeper—a co-bearer of nonlinear temporality. We hold the space in which affect returns, collapses, and refolds. We delay interpretation not because we do not know, but because we are waiting for the patient to arrive, recognizing that within the knowledge, there is also a becoming.

Conclusion—Symbolizing the Unlived

To symbolize the unlived is to make room for experience that has no place in personal narrative or cultural discourse. It is to accompany an affect that has not been named, not because it was forgotten, but because it was never given language to begin with. This is the central task of *Unstable Objects*: to trace those aspects of psychic life that do not organize easily into stories, that resist linearity, that tremble at the edges of recognition. Not as pathologies to be corrected, but as truths of experience that demand reverent presence.

We have seen, across these chapters, that the psyche is not a self-contained unit. It is a field of recursive tensions, paradoxes, fractures, and enactments. Subjectivity is not a fact, but a process; not a noun, but a verb. It is shaped not only by what has happened, but by what could not happen, by what was foreclosed, silenced, or never dreamed.

Psychic Life Beyond the Ego

Freud's vision of the ego as a mediator among drives, reality, and the superego gave way, in time, to more dynamic notions of selfhood. Loewald, Winnicott, Bion, and later relational theorists complicated the ego's sovereignty, locating psychic life in fields of co-creation and unconscious transmission. But even these expansions sometimes leaned toward integration—as if the telos of development were always wholeness.

Unstable Objects argues otherwise. Some structures are not meant to be integrated. They are meant to be held open, lived with, approached again and again. The patient who cannot speak their desire, the one who repeats without understanding, the one who dissociates at the edge of connection—these are not failed selves. They are signs of the psyche preserving itself under impossible conditions.

In this sense, psychic life extends beyond ego organization. It includes what Bollas called the "unthought known," what Ogden called "undreamt dreams," and what Eigen referred to as "depths"—affective landscapes that exist beneath formulation. These are not the unconscious as repressed content, but the unconscious as resonance: as shadowed vitality.

The Analyst as Symbolic Witness

The analytic task, then, is not to interpret our way into mastery. It is to become witnesses to the unlived. Not to extract meaning, but to offer presence. To listen without resolution. To dwell in the field of the patient's psyche as one who *stays*—not to guide, but to hold. This is not neutrality; it is attunement in its most demanding form.

We do not cure fragmentation by explaining it. We accompany it, speak to it, and become its interlocutor. We offer, in Winnicott's terms, a facilitating environment—not as a space of correction, but as a relational surround in which even the unnamable may begin to find trace-form. We symbolically hold what has not been held before.

When a patient re-enacts, the analyst's countertransference becomes a form of listening. When a patient falls silent, the analyst's patience becomes a medium for emergence. These are not techniques; they are acts of ethical presence. They say: *You may be incoherent here, and still be met*. The work is not to organize the unlived, but to give it space to unfurl, to warm in the presence of the other.

From Healing to Holding Paradox

The modern analytic aim is often framed as healing—but healing, too, can become a defense if it promises too much closure. Healing implies that there is a wound that can be sutured, a self that can be restored. But many patients come to analysis not to be restored, but to become—to symbolically arrive at aspects of self that never had a chance to emerge.

This is where paradox becomes not a philosophical idea, but an ethical stance. We work with selves who are both knowing and dissociated, both present and absent, both wave and particle. We must resist the temptation to collapse these paradoxes into coherence. Instead, we hold them long enough that the patient might begin to feel them without rupture.

To do this, the analyst must cultivate not only theoretical clarity but also emotional spaciousness. The capacity to wait, to reverberate, to be affected without demand. We do not bring the unlived into language; we make a home for it in our presence.

Recursive Narratives and Incomplete Selves

Many of the selves we encounter in clinical work are not coherent, but recursive. They loop through repetitive dynamics, haunted affects, ghosted wishes. These loops are not flaws—they are structures of survival. They are the psyche's way of staying alive when linear time fails.

We must be willing to listen to the same story again and again—not because the patient forgets, but because it is only through repetition that the story begins to change. Each telling is a symbolic re-entry. Each loop is a chance to hold what could not be held last time.

The incomplete self is not a failure of development. It is a form of truth. We do not become whole by resolving our fragmentation; we become whole by learning to bear it, to relate to it, to give it a space in the field of the other. The self is not a system—it is a site of recurrence.

Writing as Holding Environment

This book has attempted to embody the same ethics in its writing as it advocates in its theory. The prose loops, revisits, and holds paradox. It includes fragments, vignettes, and reveries. It invites the reader to linger, to pause, to be affected. It does not offer clear answers. It does not resolve. It stays.

To write psychoanalysis is not simply to explain psychic life. It is to become its scribe. To track the tremors of experience that do not yield easily to clarity. To honor the muteness that sometimes says more than speech. The page, like the analytic room, becomes a place where the unlived might stir.

What makes this difficult is that it refuses mastery. It requires us to be writers who *listen*. Who do not adorn paradox with flourish, nor rush it into explanation. We must learn to write as we analyze: with restraint, with curiosity, with love.

Symbolizing the Unlived

In the end, to symbolize the unlived is not to give it meaning, but to make it bearable. To speak it, not to solve it. To find the form through which it may flicker into view—not as revelation, but as resonance. The psyche is not a story to be told. It is a field to be inhabited.

We are all, to some extent, symbols of ourselves. Condensed, coiled, deferred. Like DNA, the self encodes futures it has not yet lived. It repeats pasts it never quite survived. It speaks in metaphor, not to be poetic, but because it must. The symbolic is not an overlay on the real—it is how the real becomes livable.

This is the hope of psychoanalysis—not to fix, not even to heal, but to live alongside. To stay near what was once unlived. To let the psyche speak in its own time, its own form, its own music. Not to hurry it. Not to decide for it. But to stay.

What else can we do, in the face of so much that resists integration, but love it into form?

11 Pathological Accommodation and the Architecture of Invisibility

This chapter re-envisions pathological accommodation not only as a structural adaptation to early misattunement, but as a recursive, aesthetic, and choreographic process—a ritualized vanishing of the self that safeguards relational bonds by suppressing affective vitality. Drawing on and extending the work of Stolorow, Atwood, and Brandchaft, I frame accommodation as a stylized sequence of relational *self-editing* that becomes both psychic architecture and ethical dilemma. Through clinical vignettes and theoretical integration, I explore how this phenomenon manifests as dissociation, curation, and performance, and how it is shaped by sociocultural demands for legibility. Rather than seeking integration or coherence, I argue that psychoanalytic presence in such treatments must emphasize restraint, aesthetic disruption, and the containment of rupture. The analytic task is not to restore authenticity, but to hold incoherence, to witness the unformulated, and to pace with the patient's own unfolding. This chapter ultimately proposes that in the treatment of pathological accommodation, transformation often arrives not through interpretation, but through eruptions of the unaccommodated self—the *beast-state*—which reorganizes the field by interrupting its choreography.

Introduction—The Quiet Violence of Becoming What Is Needed

Pathological accommodation, as originally conceptualized by Stolorow, Atwood, and Brandchaft (1994; Brandchaft et al., 2010), refers to the unconscious and recursive psychic adaptation that emerges when a child's authenticity threatens the stability of a necessary relational bond. In such cases, the developing subject learns—often pre-verbally—that the cost of presence is conditionality. One must become knowable in the language of the caregiver's emotional demands. The child responds not with protest but with compliance. Over time, this compliance is not merely behavioral, but ontological: a reconfiguration of one's being around what is emotionally tolerable to the other.

What begins as a survival strategy gradually ossifies into a relational ontology. The child does not simply *play along*—they become the self they must be in order to remain in connection. This form of accommodation is not a

DOI: 10.4324/9781003715283-15

single event, nor reducible to a defensive maneuver. It is, instead, a structure of being-in-relation—a choreography of self-displacement performed repeatedly across relational fields and often misrecognized as empathy, maturity, or attunement. It is the sacrifice of aliveness beneath the appearance of harmony.

In this chapter, I build on the intersubjective model while proposing a distinct reframing: pathological accommodation should be understood not only as a structural adaptation, but as a **ritualized temporal sequence**—a patterned, aestheticized choreography of vanishing. Through this lens, accommodation is not simply a strategy to remain in relationship, but a rehearsed disappearance that safeguards psychic coherence. It becomes a psychic performance—a way of surviving through becoming what is needed, again and again, in ways that evacuate internal experience and arrest the unfolding of affective life.

Temporality is central here. Accommodation is not a trait; it is a **sequence**, a ritual, a pacing of affective compromise that is enacted repeatedly and unconsciously. These sequences often become stylized—like a psychic routine rehearsed to perfection. Each time the subject begins to feel the stirrings of vitality, anger, eroticism, or contradiction, a familiar series of adjustments ensues: softening, anticipating, silencing, attuning. What results is not repression, but **affective curation**—a life presented in formats that are pre-cleansed of threat to the other.

This chapter also takes seriously the **aesthetic** and **ethical** dimensions of pathological accommodation. It is not enough to describe what the patient does; we must ask what kind of subjectivity emerges under relational pressure. And more challengingly, what kind of witnessing can hold such subjectivity without re-inscribing the demand for coherence, emergence, or meaning? As I will argue, the goal is not always to liberate the authentic self, but to **tolerate the opacity of survival**—to remain with the patient even when they cannot appear fully. This is a form of ethical psychoanalysis that bears witness to fragmentation without requiring its resolution.

What follows is an unfolding inquiry into the architecture of accommodation. I explore its origins, its recursive forms, and its aesthetic strategies. I draw on a range of theorists—Stolorow, Brandchaft, Bromberg, Benjamin, Mitchell, Ogden, Harris, Butler, and others—to develop a clinical and theoretical vocabulary for psychic performances that are exquisitely crafted yet hollowed from within. Ultimately, I ask what kind of analytic presence can hold what has been repeatedly made to vanish. And whether, in certain moments, it is not working through but **rupture**—an emergence of something beastly, erotic, incoherent, and real—that reorganizes the field in ways that no interpretation can.

Theoretical Foundations—Patterns of Survival, Not Traits

Stolorow, Atwood, and Brandchaft's (1994) intersubjective theory of development provides a crucial lens for understanding the nonvolitional origins of pathological accommodation. Their original formulation already emphasizes the recursive and temporally layered nature of relational life. Temporality is not an add-on to their framework—it is embedded in the very idea that the self takes shape through repeated affective encounters. The psyche, in this view, is not formed in isolation but sculpted across time by the emotional fields it inhabits.

My aim here is not to introduce temporality into the concept of accommodation, but to extend and aestheticize it. I propose that accommodation is best understood not simply as an internalized relational compromise, but as a stylized sequence of psychic adjustments—a choreography of vanishing that becomes structural through recursive enactment. These sequences are not incidental. They become internal architecture: repeated scenes of survival performed so seamlessly that they come to resemble character.

The child whose vitality disrupts the field learns to modulate not only their behavior but also their affect. What begins as adaptation becomes habituated stylization. The developing subject may not repress feeling, but learn to delay it, dress it, soften it—transforming raw affect into something palatable. Over time, this yields a relational aesthetic in which the self is always slightly edited, always paced according to what can be borne by the other.

Borrowing from Alfred Lorenzer's (1981) concept of scenic understanding, we can view pathological accommodation as composed of such stylized scenes: internalized relational dramas in which the subject plays a rehearsed role—the softened one, the helpful one, the non-disruptive presence. These scenes are not remembered; they are lived. The patient may unconsciously pace speech, attenuate affect, or offer insight in just the right rhythm to be well received. What appears as fluency is often a ritual. What seems like maturity may be a choreography of evasion. The self becomes not simply adaptive, but curated.

These aestheticized patterns are often mistaken for relational skill. The patient may present as empathic, emotionally intelligent, even precociously attuned. But underneath the fluency is an overtranslation of inner life: a stylized effort to ensure psychic safety through coherence. Over time, this coherence becomes hollow. The patient survives—but not as themselves.

Clinical Illustration: Ethan

My patient, Ethan, was a high-functioning man in his early thirties who came to treatment describing a vague dissatisfaction with his relationships. He had no explicit complaints—he was successful, in a stable partnership, and socially embedded. What he could not describe, though, was a feeling of inhabiting his life. He said it felt "like performing a version of myself that works, but isn't quite mine."

Our early sessions were marked by grace. Ethan was deeply attuned, articulate, even lyrical in his reflections. He anticipated my responses, offered self-insights, and always arrived having already metabolized his week's events. I noticed how often I left our sessions feeling effective, even idealized. And yet, a strange flatness persisted—a sense that something essential was always slightly out of reach.

Over time, I began to notice how his narratives arrived pre-digested. There was very little raw affect, even when he described painful or disorienting events. When I gently inquired into his emotional experience, he would offer beautiful reflections, but rarely direct feelings. My interpretations were received warmly, even gratefully, but they never seemed to shift anything. The therapy was smooth, curated—and increasingly unalive.

One afternoon, I asked him to pause mid-narrative and simply notice what he was feeling in his body. He fell silent. Then, almost imperceptibly, his face changed. His eyes narrowed. He said, very quietly, "I hate this." I asked what he hated. "This," he said again. "The way I'm talking to you. The way I already know what you're going to say. The way I'm trying to make this work so you don't think I'm wasting your time."

He looked shocked. I said nothing.

He went on, more agitated now. "You're good at this. You say good things. But I think I hate how much I want you to like me." He paused. "I'm so tired of shaping myself around people who don't even ask for it."

This was a rupture. Not rage, exactly, but a rupture in the rhythm of our aesthetic contract. A raw refusal, a confession not of insight but of exhaustion. Something uncurated had appeared. It was not an insight to be interpreted, but a truth to be honored.

I said simply, "I believe you."

We sat in silence for several minutes. He did not try to soften what he had said. I did not try to respond with depth. What passed between us was not a formulation, but a holding—a shared exposure to what had previously been impossible to feel in the room. The choreography of accommodation had faltered. And in its absence, something flickered: not a new self, but a field less governed by performance.

In this early rupture, Ethan's beast-state revealed not a hidden truth, but a destabilized pattern. What followed was not narrative integration, but the slow capacity to remain near what could not yet be named.

This section reframes pathological accommodation as a ritualized, temporally embedded aesthetic—a survival choreography mistaken for character. In the next section, I turn to the dissociative residues this choreography leaves in its wake: the internal voids, the sequestered affect, and the fragmented time-sense that haunt even the most fluent presentations of self.

Fragmentation and Dissociation—From Alien Self to Splintered Time

The recursive performance of pathological accommodation fractures internal experience in ways that may not initially appear dissociative. Unlike classic trauma-based dissociation, which often severs consciousness from overwhelming experience, accommodation operates more subtly. It does not obliterate parts of the self; it renders them inadmissible. Over time, the subject does not forget what they feel—they simply lose access to the internal conditions that would allow those feelings to emerge without disorganizing the relational field.

Brandchaft's concept of the "alien self system" (2010) captures part of this phenomenon. In the service of survival, the patient builds an internal structure not to deceive but to remain included. This alien self is not false in the pejorative sense. It is exquisitely attuned to the demands of the relational surround. Yet beneath its functionality, other affective states—rage, joy, erotic intensity, grief—are sequestered, unavailable, or only partially known.

Bromberg (1998) helps us understand how this sequestering is not merely repressive but **dissociative**. The patient who accommodates is often living in **a narrowed field of permissible self-states**, with others cordoned off as unlivable or dangerous. These sequestered states may return in the form of somatic symptoms, dissociative fog, erotic enactments, or unaccountable affect storms. Yet even their return may be met with re-accommodation: the patient soothes, censors, or performs over them in order to maintain coherence. Unlike trauma-based dissociation, which fractures consciousness through psychic overwhelm, accommodation-based dissociation fragments affect through stylization. It is not the obliteration of self, but the recursive rehearsal of admissible self-states.

What emerges is not fragmentation as collapse, but fragmentation as performance. The patient is not split in the classical sense—they are dispersed across stylized self-states, inhabiting a curated surface calibrated for smoothness, empathy, and fluency. Yet the cost of such fluency is affective discontinuity. Aesthetic coherence becomes the mask over a dissociated interior.

Donnel Stern (2003) offers the concept of the unformulated experience—experience that exists but has not been symbolized. In pathological accommodation, much of psychic life remains unformulated, not because it lacks intensity, but because it has never had a relational context in which it could be metabolized. These unformulated experiences linger beneath the surface of the stylized self, creating a pressure that can feel like anxiety, shame, or dread when proximity to authenticity threatens to rupture the curated form.

Adrienne Harris (2005) and Muriel Dimen (2003) expand our understanding by showing how these dynamics are shaped by cultural scripts of gender, race, and power. The demand to appear coherent, pleasing, or emotionally available is not evenly distributed. Women, queer people, and racialized subjects are often required to develop precocious emotional labor capacities in order to remain safe or included. In such cases, accommodation is not only interpersonal—it is political. The fragmentation it installs is not simply psychic, but **culturally scaffolded**.

This dissociative compartmentalization was especially evident in another patient, Luis, a graduate student in literature who appeared to live entirely in a register of refined insight. Each session began with eloquent interpretations of his dreams, reflections on recent readings, or philosophical musings on the analytic process itself. What was absent was affect. Despite his intelligence and insight, his emotional presence in the room felt spectral, as though we were always speaking about experience, never from within it.

I remember a session where he narrated a recent breakup in meticulous psychological and theoretical detail. He named every defense mechanism he had likely employed. But when I asked how the breakup had felt in his body, he blinked. There was a long pause. Then he said, "Oh. That's a different register, isn't it?" He tried, briefly, to locate sensation—his throat, he said, had felt tight—but abandoned the effort quickly and returned to narrating his partner's probable attachment style.

This wasn't resistance. It was a ritual. The return to theoretical distance was part of a choreography that had long protected Luis from emotional exposure. He could be exquisite in his self-awareness but absent from his own pain. In his case, dissociation didn't appear as forgetting or blankness—it appeared as brilliance. As in Ethan's case, the dissociative structure was not a retreat from meaning, but a performance of legibility so total that it had overwritten the body's raw signals. These are not patients who are cut off from themselves in a classical sense. Rather, they are **haunted by a self they have learned to avoid becoming**.

This fragmentation is not a failure of integration, but a survival logic within a world that cannot receive the full range of the subject's being. In the clinic, such patients may present as insightful and emotionally articulate, yet struggle with a persistent sense of inauthenticity. They may describe a life that functions but does not feel lived. The work, then, is not to interpret their symptoms as repressed truths, but to understand their suffering as the residue of dissociation that is structured, repeated, and reinforced by both developmental and ongoing relational demands.

In the next section, I turn to the aesthetic strategies by which this fragmentation is covered over—not only for others, but often for the patient themselves. Through the lens of curation, performance, and the false self, we see how dissociation is rendered legible, even beautiful—at the cost of aliveness.

Aesthetic Survival—Curation as Psychic Strategy

If the dissociation inherent in pathological accommodation creates gaps, then aesthetic coherence fills them. The curated self is not merely an artifact of trauma or misattunement—it is a deliberate survival structure, one that cloaks fragmentation beneath fluency. This aesthetic coherence, often experienced by clinicians as likability, charisma, empathy, or refinement, conceals the deeper truth: a self that has been crafted rather than emerged.

Here, the false self is not a mask in the traditional Winnicottian sense, nor merely a defensive posture. It is a living installation—an emotional and interpersonal design that anticipates, soothes, and reflects the needs of others before they are spoken. This self does not lie. It reveals selectively. It edits.

To understand this form of accommodation as a **curatorial act** is to recognize its intentionality. Not conscious intention, but a layered, recursive intelligence—a choreography of omission, modulation, and substitution that turns raw affect into palatable gesture. The subject does not perform badly; they perform exquisitely. Their pain, if it is offered at all, is metabolized for the viewer. Their shame is repackaged as sensitivity. Their eroticism is translated into allure. It is a kind of psychic design, aimed not only at being received but also praised.

This is the false self, not as a lie, but as a **relational aesthetic**. It is the shape the self takes when it must always be both object and mirror. A curation of coherence in the face of disintegration. This dynamic is especially visible in patients who appear deeply empathic, intuitive, and relationally skilled—whose very attunement to the analyst masks the absence of internal attunement to themselves.

Judith Butler's (2005) work on recognition helps illuminate the sociopolitical context in which this curation occurs. To be recognized, one must become recognizable. Psychic life becomes formatted for consumption—its intelligibility measured not by its authenticity, but by its legibility within shared social and relational codes. Foucault (1977) calls this the production of the docile body—shaped not by overt force but by internalized surveillance. In psychic terms, this results in the self that watches itself from within, arranging its display to maintain coherence in the face of exposure.

Dimen's (2003) writing on the erotics of submission and Adrienne Harris's (2005) work on multiplicity both reveal how this form of psychic curation is often imbued with both necessity and desire. The curated self becomes not only a safety measure but also a source of identity—especially for those whose early environments made spontaneity dangerous or invisibility intolerable. As a result, the patient may feel both resentment toward and identification with the false self. It has protected them, but it has also prevented them.

Bracha Ettinger (2006) offers a potential counterpoint. In her work on the matrixial borderspace, she imagines a form of subjectivity that is neither entirely separate nor entirely fused—a co-emergent field where fragility and presence coexist. Through this lens, one might imagine a patient's curated self not as a betrayal of emergence, but as its wounded residue: a self born into a field that could not hold its incoherence, and so became stylized to survive.

Importantly, the analyst is also invited into the aesthetic. The well-curated patient often pulls the analyst into admiration, collusion, or even envy. These are the patients analysts often describe as "a pleasure to work with"—insightful, articulate, self-aware. Yet this pleasure may mask a collusion with invisibility. The analyst may unconsciously reward the very performance that protects the patient from feeling.

But the countertransference may also be more complex than admiration or aesthetic collusion. With some patients, the curated presence elicits not pleasure but unease—a subtle sense of dislocation or fatigue in the analyst. I have found myself, in such treatments, feeling intermittently effective and irrelevant, welcomed and kept at bay. There is often a strange clarity in the hour, paired with a mysterious absence of impact. These patients may evoke not only gratitude for their self-reflection but also a nagging sense that the session never quite happened.

This disorientation is itself instructive. It marks the analyst's encounter with a psychic surface that is too smooth to grip. There is little traction. The feeling of being gently repelled—of being included in the patient's aesthetic but excluded from their interior—is often the first clue that we are not simply in the presence of emotional maturity, but of a survival structure polished to brilliance. In such moments, the analyst's task is not to push through, but to notice the form: to become attuned to the rhythm of the accommodation itself and to resist the pull to either idealize or interrogate.

Clinical Illustration: Julian

Julian was a patient in his late thirties who worked in a design-related field and carried himself with remarkable poise. From the beginning of our work, I found myself struck by his precision—not only in language but also in affect. His speech was polished, considered, and often beautiful. He offered scenes from his life with just enough vulnerability to create emotional resonance, but rarely lingered in the rawness of any moment.

He frequently framed emotional pain in metaphor: "It's like a gallery that's been carefully lit—you see the shape of the thing, but never the heat." These metaphors were evocative, even moving, but I began to sense that they arrived preassembled. I felt I was being handed artful fragments rather than encountering someone from within.

Over time, I noticed how easily I was pulled into admiration. Julian's insights were sophisticated, his relational awareness acute. But the very ease of our sessions began to trouble me. I would leave our meetings with a nagging sense that nothing had quite happened—no rupture, no friction, no moment of genuine encounter. The therapy was exquisite, but uninhabited.

One day, after Julian shared a story about a recent conflict with a colleague—one he described with calm detachment and even generosity—I said gently, "I wonder how it felt to be in that moment, not just to describe it." He paused, looked down, and said, "I'm not sure I know how to answer that. I can give you the shape of what happened, but I think I edited the part of me that felt it."

Then, almost apologetically, he added, "I've always been good at packaging things. It's how I stay… safe, I think."

That moment shifted the field. What had felt like resistance revealed itself as ritual. His aesthetic fluency was not a flourish—it was a survival strategy, a way of staying visible while remaining untouched.

From then on, our work took a different course. Julian began to notice his own stylization in real time. He would sometimes pause mid-sentence and say, "That was the curated version—let me try again." Often, he could not.

But the pause itself became meaningful. We had entered a space where the performance could falter without needing to be replaced.

My countertransference in this work was subtle but instructive. I felt both privileged and peripheral—welcomed, yet somehow irrelevant. It became clear that I was being positioned not as an interlocutor but as an audience. The session had become a stage, and Julian its only actor. My task, then, was not to dismantle the performance, but to remain near it—to notice its rhythms, to hear its edges soften, and to resist the temptation to interpret too soon.

Julian's accommodation was not dramatic, but it was complete. It shaped his speech, his silences, and his ability to predict the emotional needs of others. And when the ritual occasionally frayed—when his voice cracked, when he didn't know what to say—something unpracticed flickered in. Not a revelation. A presence.

Ethical Complexity—Witnessing without Demanding Emergence

Psychoanalysis has long been oriented around the value of emergence. The movement from dissociation to integration, from symptom to symbol, from alien self to authentic subjectivity—these are the familiar arcs of the analytic process. Yet for patients whose inner lives have been formed through chronic accommodation, the call to emerge may echo the very relational violence they seek to escape. What appears as therapeutic encouragement can quickly become another demand: be more real, be more whole, be more visible.

In this section, I argue that the treatment of pathological accommodation requires a distinct ethical posture—one that is not organized around revelation or coherence, but around the discipline of **non-demanding presence**. This presence does not ask the patient to appear more fully, but stays near their opacity, their hesitation, their incoherence. It resists the temptation to rescue, decode, or assemble. Instead, it witnesses.

Stolorow and Brandchaft (2010) describe analytic healing in terms of emancipation—the freeing of the self from alien structures that no longer serve it. This remains a powerful ideal. Yet if emancipation is structured around legibility, it risks reinscribing the core wound of accommodation. The demand to become legible—even to the analyst—can replicate the demand to be someone else's version of real. For patients whose survival has been organized around knowing what the other needs, even well-meaning recognition may feel like a violation.

Emmanuel Levinas (1969) offers a philosophical alternative. For Levinas, ethics does not begin with understanding the other, but with honoring the other's unknowability. The ethical relationship is one in which the self does not consume the other as an object of knowledge, but sustains their alterity. Applied clinically, this suggests that the analyst's task is not to make the patient more comprehensible, but to remain present to their unintelligibility. To bear witness not to what is revealed, but to what resists revelation.

Jessica Benjamin (2004) similarly invites us to consider the analyst's role not as knower but as co-participant in a relational third. The goal is not to reflect the patient back to themselves, nor to stand in opposition, but to create a space in which the patient might begin to feel real without having to perform reality. This thirdness depends not on resonance, but on *restraint*. It is the refusal to foreclose the field of potentiality with premature understanding.

Donna Orange (2010) speaks of empathy as an ethical act—not a mirroring, but a being-with. In cases of pathological accommodation, empathy must not slide into interpretation. The analyst must tolerate the patient's absence, fragmentation, and incoherence and avoid translating these states as narrative too soon. To do so risks collapsing the ritual of survival into a symptom to be treated, rather than a truth to be held.

This ethic of restraint becomes even more vital when we consider the sociopolitical scaffolding of accommodation. Frantz Fanon (1967/1952) and Sylvia Wynter (2003) both articulate how subjectivity is shaped by dominant norms of legibility. To be Black, queer, feminine, or otherwise marked is to be pressured into appearing coherent, respectable, intelligible—on someone else's terms. In this light, accommodation is not only a developmental compromise but a **social demand**, and one that carries intergenerational weight.

The social dimension of legibility came sharply into focus with my patient Darius, a queer Black man in his late twenties, who described his life as a series of rehearsals. "I'm always previewing myself," he said. "Even when I'm alone, there's a kind of imagined watcher I'm trying to manage." He had learned to offer what he called "the polished pain"—just enough vulnerability to seem real, but never enough to risk rejection. In our work, this dynamic repeated itself. Darius would deliver fragments of his history in beautifully structured monologues, carefully modulated, often accompanied by a self-deprecating laugh.

When I asked how it felt to be that composed while speaking of intimate loss, he said, "I don't get to just feel things. I have to translate them for white people." That sentence landed with a quiet force, reorienting the room and reframing the terms of our contact. It reframed his aesthetic fluency not as a defense, but as survival choreography within a racialized field of demand. His accommodation was not only personal—it was **politically inherited**.

Fanon (1967/1952) described this internalization as "epidermalization"—the implantation of the colonizer's gaze beneath the skin. Wynter (2003) extends this critique by insisting that the very idea of the "fully human" is shaped by coloniality. For patients like Darius, then, the therapeutic invitation to "be yourself" may echo historical violences. Emergence is not simply difficult—it can feel like exposure to a gaze that has always already misread you. Witnessing, in such cases, cannot be neutral. It must include an awareness of the analyst's own positionality—and a willingness to **forgo recognition as the ethical aim**.

Darius's disclosure reframed the stakes of analytic witnessing. What may appear as avoidance or stylization may, in fact, be the most authentic offering a patient can make within a structure of inherited scrutiny. The clinician, then, must take care not to confuse incoherence with resistance or performance with evasion. The task is not to extract what is hidden, but to remain with what is only partially visible—and to sit beside the patient's curated presence, asking not what lies behind it, but what it costs to keep it up.

This stance is not passive. It is deeply active in its restraint. It involves the constant discipline of resisting interpretive closure, of holding open the space of potentiality, and of listening for what is not said—not in order to decode it, but to acknowledge its right to remain unspeakable.

This form of witnessing can be quietly transformative. When the patient senses that their analyst does not require them to be real in a particular way, something loosens. The pressure to curate softens. The choreography of accommodation may falter. And in that faltering, the analytic field may begin to tremble with something more alive—something not yet known, not yet shown, but suddenly possible.

In the next section, I turn toward these ruptural moments as sites of radical transformation—not because they reveal what has been hidden, but because they **interrupt the choreography itself**, offering an uncurated glimpse of being that can reorganize the field without demanding coherence.

The Royal Road to the Real—Working Through and Reorganizing Ruptures

Freud famously called dreams "the royal road to the unconscious," suggesting that even distorted psychic material could offer symbolic access to the truths of inner life. In contemporary analytic practice—particularly in the treatment of patients organized around pathological accommodation—we might ask whether a parallel royal road exists. Not one that leads to the unconscious through metaphor, but one that leads to the real—that which resists symbolization altogether.

For these patients, it is not the dream, but the rupture—the moment when choreography fails, when the softened register collapses—that offers the most direct encounter with the unspeakable core of psychic life. The analytic field is often marked by a rhythm of anticipation and disappearance, in which vitality is suppressed before it can be felt. But occasionally, something breaks through. A flicker of unsoftened affect. A moment of erotic intensity. An act of refusal or contempt. These are not narrative revelations; they are ruptures in form—eruptions of a self that has not been accommodated.

Working through remains vital. It allows for interpretation, meaning-making, and narrative reconstruction. It can help loosen the grip of accommodation by locating it historically and affectively. But for some patients, especially those whose survival has required exquisite modulation of affect and expression, interpretation may come second to presence. For them, reorganization may not come through insight, but through rupture—a break in the ritual, a moment when the choreography collapses.

These are the moments when what Bollas (1987) calls the "true self" announces itself—not through verbal insight, but through discontinuity. Eigen

(2004) might call this the pulse of being: a raw, affective state that is unformed, unfiltered, and yet unmistakably alive. It is the moment the analyst does not expect, cannot explain, and must not interrupt. Ogden (1994) reminds us that the analyst must often endure what is "not yet thinkable"—not to push it into formulation, but to keep it company in its pre-symbolic state.

Stephen Mitchell (1988) offers a particularly generative metaphor for this process. In *Relational Concepts in Psychoanalysis*, he describes the "beast" as the affectively charged, unruly, and disruptive presence that lurks beneath the smooth surface of relational form. This beast is not pathological. It is vital. It is the part of the self that resists domestication. For patients steeped in accommodation, the beast is what they have had to hide, modulate, or transform into something consumable. Its emergence in the analytic space is not a regression, but a breakthrough.

We can build on Mitchell's framing to propose that the **beast-state** is the counterpoint to accommodation. If accommodation is a stylized repetition of legible selfhood, then the beast is its rupture. A burst of affect, desire, or incoherence that interrupts the psychic routine. These moments do not need to be interpreted; they need to be held. Their power lies in their refusal to be smoothed.

Some patients may blurt something hostile mid-session, then immediately apologize. Others may go suddenly silent, drop eye contact, or dissociate in a way that breaks the rhythm of their usual coherence. Still others may weep without narrative or enter the session caught in a charged intensity they themselves cannot make sense of. These moments often do not resolve—they destabilize. And it is in the destabilization that something reorganizes, not in terms of clarity or catharsis, but in terms of permission: a moment where what is usually foreclosed is permitted to appear, however briefly.

Rather than positioning working through and rupture as opposites, this chapter frames them as twin pathways—interpretation and eruption—that together contour the topography of transformation. A flicker of the beast-state—a gasp, a flash of contempt, a flooded erotic moment—may not be narratively elaborated, nor require symbolization to be meaningful. These are not moments to be resolved, but to be witnessed without taming.

The emergence of the beast does not always lend itself to interpretation. It cuts through. And in doing so, it performs a kind of reorganization not through insight, but through interruption. These moments often carry an unexpected integrity: the patient does not need to explain or even understand what has broken through. They need only to survive being in it, with the analyst staying close, not pulling the moment back into coherence. This is not the linear arc of working through, but a circular flash—a return of what has been exiled, pulsing with a form of vitality that does not ask permission.

As Mitchell suggests, the beast may emerge in psychoanalysis not as a primitive vestige to be tamed, but as a destabilizing excess that exposes the limits of relational form. In moments when the patient's accommodation falters—when the usual sequence of pleasing, softening, or foreclosing is interrupted—what appears may not be a new self, but something older and less linguistically mediated. Erotic, feral, or dissociated, this beast-state cannot be organized through mutuality; it resists interpretation and threatens coherence. And yet, it is often in the wake of such ruptures that the analytic field begins to reconfigure, no longer governed solely by survival choreography but by the pulse of something unmastered. These states may mark not a breakdown, but a bid—however inchoate—for aliveness outside the rituals of appeasement.

In this light, working through and holding reorganizing ruptures are not opposed but parallel forms of analytic care. One unfolds through words; the other through presence. One moves through insight and interpretation; the other halts, surrounds, and contains. Both are royal roads. But the latter leads not to interpretation, but to the Real—that Lacanian excess, that Eigenian pulse, that Bollasian emergence of the unthought known. In the context of pathological accommodation, where performance has replaced presence, it may be these beastly ruptures that most fully return the patient to themselves.

Clinical Vignette and Reflection

The following clinical vignette illustrates the psychic architecture of pathological accommodation and the transformative potential of rupture when held rather than interpreted. Names and identifying details have been changed.

My patient, Clara, was a queer woman in her early forties who entered treatment describing a general sense of "unreality" in her relationships. She was an artist and educator, known for her generosity and perceptiveness, but described herself as "someone people open up to, but rarely look at." Her life, while outwardly full, felt to her like a sequence of offerings: attention, care, attunement—rarely returned in kind. "I think I just became good at making space for other people's realities," she said in an early session. "Eventually, I forgot I had one."

Clara was thoughtful, articulate, and often moved quickly to explore emotional dynamics. But something in the room remained elusive. Each session felt luminous but untethered. Even as she offered evocative material, she seemed unlocatable inside it. When I asked how particular stories or interactions had felt to her, she would often answer with insight or with a story about how someone else had felt. There was always a narrative—graceful, pre-digested—but rarely a pulse.

After several months, I found myself feeling increasingly ineffective. Our sessions were intimate, textured, even poignant, but I began leaving them with a strange fatigue—as if I had been kept close, but not quite permitted entry. One day, after she described a conflict with a close friend in polished and empathic terms, I said softly, "I notice how carefully you've located everyone else's experience. I wonder where yours is."

Clara paused. Her face changed—not in defensiveness, but in something like collapse. "That's the thing," she said. "I don't think I'm allowed to have one. Or maybe I don't know how to stay with it. It's like—if I feel something too much, I won't be able to make space for them. And then they'll leave."

I said nothing. She looked down and added, "Sometimes I think my feelings are dangerous just for existing."

This was the rupture—not dramatic, but quietly searing. A flicker of the beast-state in its most tender form: not rage, not eruption, but the emergence of a nearly unspeakable conviction that presence itself was unsafe. Her narrative hadn't shifted, but the field had. What appeared in that moment wasn't content—it was proximity.

From then on, our work became slower. Clara began noticing how quickly she pre-processed her emotional life. "I can feel myself putting it through the softening machine," she once said. "Before it even gets to you." There were times she would stop mid-story, close her eyes, and say, "Wait—let me try again. That version was for someone else."

These moments were not cathartic; they were disorienting, painful, and occasionally silent. But they were alive. The choreography had faltered, and in its faltering, something began to cohere—not a self, necessarily, but a field that could hold what had once been pre-emptively dissolved.

What this clinical process illuminated most starkly was the aesthetic elegance with which Clara had survived. Her curated self was not defensive—it was devotional. A life organized around making room for others while quietly displacing herself. The beast-state, in her case, was not a roar but a whisper: a sentence, a pause, a refusal to translate.

My task was not to interpret these flickers, nor to encourage their continuity. It was to endure them. To notice when the softened version arrived and wait patiently to see if a different one might emerge. And to respect the fact that sometimes, it wouldn't.

Pathological accommodation does not always announce itself in suffering. It arrives in grace, in insight, in unshakable relational fluency. But beneath it, there may be a ritual of disappearance so complete that even the patient cannot locate its beginnings. When the ritual falters—when something less presentable appears—the analytic space can become something else entirely: not a mirror, not a stage, but a witness to what was never supposed to arrive.

Conclusion—Psychic Survival, Uncohered, and Held

Clara's flickering self-presence—tentative, partial, and sometimes vanishing—offers a final window into the nature of pathological accommodation. What these treatments reveal is not merely a structure of avoidance, but a lived, temporal choreography: a psychic aesthetic crafted to prevent abandonment by pre-empting emergence. In such lives, presence is not simply delayed—it is repackaged, stylized, softened until it disappears. The analyst's work is not to unveil what is hidden, but to remain near what has been rehearsed into nonexistence.

Pathological accommodation is often mistaken for a relational strength. Its fluency, empathy, and attunement are easy to admire. But beneath the aesthetic coherence lies a recursive ritual of vanishing—a survival strategy that substitutes performative selfhood for affective presence. In this chapter, I have argued that accommodation is not merely a response to early misattunement, but a temporal, choreographic phenomenon: a stylized sequence of emotional adjustments that keeps the self safely legible at the cost of vitality.

Such survival is not failure. It is brilliance forged in the face of ongoing psychic and social demand. To pathologize accommodation is to miss its ethical weight. These are patients who have built lives—beautiful, competent, relational lives—while systematically subtracting themselves from them. The cost is not always obvious. But in the analytic room, it emerges as dissociation, curation, over-translation, and a haunting sense of unreality.

I have sought to reframe our clinical task with these patients. Not to extract the true self, nor to interpret every silence, but to bear witness to the ritual itself—to the choreography of accommodation as a lived structure. I have suggested that ethical psychoanalysis in these cases depends on the analyst's capacity to **stay with incoherence**—to honor opacity, fragmentation, and aesthetic defense without requiring their resolution. This is a discipline of restraint, and one that carries its own psychic risks.

In certain moments, the ritual falters. And in that faltering, something appears—not a new self, but the beast-state: an eruption of unaccommodated being that may be erotic, affectively jagged, or incoherent. These moments are not always narratable. They do not ask to be interpreted. They ask to be **held**. This holding is not passive. It is a stance of deep ethical engagement, in which the analyst declines the familiar reward of meaning in favor of presence.

We might say that psychoanalysis, at its best, makes room for lives that have not yet been lived. But in cases of pathological accommodation, the work may be less about living forward and more about staying near what has never been able to arrive—what has always been pre-emptively softened, stylized, or erased.

To do this requires a shift in our clinical values. From integration to interruption. From legibility to witnessing. From emergence to **endurance**. The patient may never fully abandon their choreography. Nor must they. But the analytic space can become one of quiet disobedience—where the curated self need not be dismantled to be seen, and where moments of rupture are not feared, but recognized as **the royal road to the real.**

In this sense, the work of undoing accommodation is not unlike mourning—not of a single loss, but of the unlived. The analyst and patient together grieve what could not be felt, what had to be softened before it could arrive. The silence around certain affects is not empty; it is saturated with the weight of what has been rehearsed into disappearance. And when the choreography breaks, what emerges may be jagged, incomplete, or unbearably tender. To remain with that tenderness—without naming it too quickly—is a form of mourning that resists closure.

But this mourning is not without futurity. In the analytic space, even fragments may point forward. A flicker of resentment, a subtle refusal, the unexpected emergence of erotic charge—each may rupture the smooth surface of the curated self and signal a pulse of desire not yet organized. These moments are not revelations; they are invitations. Not to interpret, but to stay. To witness. To refuse the return to coherence.

The analytic task is not to restore the real self, nor to demolish the false one, but to sit beside the oscillation—to hear the pulse in the performance, the echo in the silence, the grief in the grace. When this is done with rigor and restraint, the field itself undergoes a shift. Not into wholeness, but into **possibility**. A future that does not require the patient to be anything other than what they are: present, incoherent, flickering—and still alive.

It is tempting, in analytic work, to gather meaning quickly—to name, interpret, or claim insight before the patient's expression has fully arrived. But in cases of pathological accommodation, timing is everything. What emerges in the analytic space may not be ready to be understood. A moment of rupture—a flicker of anger, a confusing erotic pull, a withdrawal—may be less a disclosure than a test: not of interpretation, but of containment.

Patients whose lives have required constant calibration to others often approach authenticity with caution. The analytic space becomes a field not only of potential freedom, but of anticipated recapture. In this light, to hold a moment without harvesting it is a form of radical accompaniment. Not passive. Not inert. But active in its refusal to turn the patient's flicker of aliveness into a narrative that belongs to the analyst.

The deeper ethic here is temporal. Some forms of truth cannot be asked for. They arrive when the choreography falters and are sustained only if they are not pursued. The analyst's discipline, then, is to pace with the patient's capacity for emergence—not to lead it. To accompany the rhythms of survival until the patient, in their own time, lets something uncurated appear—and waits to see if we can bear it.

Symbolic Lexicon

A Living Vocabulary of Paradox, Process, and Symbolic Life

Beast-State: The sequestered drive-state that forms beneath polished psychic adaptations. Often shadowing pathological accommodation, the *Beast-State* is saturated, under-symbolized, and sometimes erotic. It does not appear as a coherent part of the self, but as a visceral leak—rage, hunger, sexual demand, annihilation fantasy. It is neither "authentic self" nor pathology, but a concentrated remainder, where aliveness pulses beneath the choreography. The analyst's task is not to tame the beast, but to witness its meaning.

Clinical Spiral: The nonlinear movement of the analytic process through recursive returns. Material re-emerges not as repetition compulsion but as *symbolic spiraling*—each return is altered, refracted, thickened. The Clinical Spiral resists the fantasy of progress. Instead of a trajectory toward resolution, it enacts something like symbolic accretion: the same image now freighted with new tone, new tension. To follow the spiral is to track transformation without destination.

Defenses Against Aliveness: Not all defenses ward off pain. Some protect against *aliveness*. This includes the unbearable intimacy of being seen, the threat of joy, and the vertigo of affective intensity. These defenses often appear as inhibition, aestheticization, or a flattened self-presentation. They may manifest as intellectualization, dissociation, or even manic pleasure. The analyst must tread carefully here: aliveness is not always welcome. To feel fully may also mean to come undone.

Disorganizing Truth: Truth that destabilizes more than it clarifies. Some insights do not integrate—they unmoor. These are not false, but *too real*: they arrive before the psyche has a structure to contain them. Disorganizing truth may emerge in trauma recovery, erotic transference, or aesthetic shock. It threatens the known self. The analyst must tread lightly here, not rushing to metabolize, but offering symbolic companionship while the psyche reorganizes in response to the impact.

Erotic Submission: More than masochism, less than surrender, erotic submission is a psychic and symbolic choreography. It stages a paradox: the subject enacts power by giving it away, finds safety in being undone, and locates selfhood in the act of being temporarily erased. Clinically, it may appear as sexual enactment, relational regression, or transferential positioning. Its function is not defensive but *ritualistic*—a symbolic rehearsal of annihilation, contact, and symbolic rebirth.

Ethical Refusal: A form of psychic resistance in which the subject declines to participate in a relational or symbolic process that feels prematurely imposed, developmentally untimely, or affectively unsafe. Unlike defensive withdrawal, *Ethical Refusal* is not a retreat from meaning but a principled suspension of it—a refusal to be known before the conditions of recognition are ethically sound. It may manifest as dissociative stillness, fragmented narrative, or affective delay, particularly in analytic contexts where the demand for coherence risks recapitulating earlier intrusions. *Ethical Refusal* honors the psychic integrity of the unformed or unborn self, signaling not pathology but fidelity to a truth that has not yet found symbolic hospitality. In this sense, it reflects a paradoxical vitality: a refusal to collapse into legibility when legibility would violate the soul's timing. For the analyst, it calls for a stance of disciplined receptivity—a willingness to wait, to unknow, and to offer coherence only after containment has done its necessary, wordless work.

False Self as Curator: A reframing of Winnicott's False Self not as merely defensive, but as *aesthetic*. The false self becomes a curator—organizing the self as a collection, performance, and symbolic scaffold. This curator does not lie; it arranges. It maintains relational coherence by displaying what others can bear. The cost is not falseness but alienation from the unspeakable object within.

Fragmented Witnessing: A form of presence that does not require coherence. Fragmented witnessing allows the analyst to remain with what cannot yet be integrated—affect that floods or slips, images without sequence, truths without grammar. It contrasts with the fantasy of "holding it all." This is not failure, but fidelity: to witness without resolving, to attune without imposing narrative.

Held Collapse: The state in which psychic fragmentation is not resolved but witnessed. Collapse here is not a breakdown in the pathological sense, but a momentary folding—of coherence, of continuity, of self-narrative. To hold collapse means neither to fix nor to interpret it, but to remain symbolically present while the patient's structure softens or slips. Held Collapse marks a rupture that does not lead to retraumatization, but to symbolic possibility.

Internal Secrecy: Not what is kept from others, but what is kept from oneself by way of survival. Internal secrecy is the structure that allows the psyche to live with contradiction—to preserve the unbearable by cordoning it off with symbolic elegance or dissociative distance. Often mistaken for repression or resistance, internal secrecy is a kind of inner architecture. In analysis, the work is not to expose the secret, but to come close without collapse.

Original Paradox: The primal contradiction at the root of psychic life: that to become a subject, one must split. The Original Paradox appears across myths, drives, and theory: to be known is to be exposed; to connect is to risk dissolution; to symbolize is to lose what was symbolized. It echoes Klein's splitting, Bion's unmentalized beta-elements, and Gödel's incompleteness: the psyche forms itself *at the site of its own impossibility*.

Partial Integration: A state of psychic organization that is not whole, but alive. Partial integration allows for complexity, contradiction, and symbolic reverberation without demanding full resolution. It resists the binary of fragmentation versus cohesion. In many patients—especially those with histories of relational trauma—this is the most stable and generative structure available.

Pathological Accommodation: Not mere submission to the other's needs, but an identity structured around anticipatory erasure. The self is not simply compliant—it is performed through invisible labor designed to sustain others' coherence. In this framing, pathology is not in accommodation per se, but in the foreclosure of symbolic alternatives. True accommodation becomes pathological when it disallows interruption, rupture, or opacity.

Psychic Remainder: What cannot be said, not because it is repressed, but because it resists symbolization altogether. The psychic remainder is what lingers after working-through, after insight, after narrative. It may be a look, a pause, a residue of tension in the analytic room. The remainder is not noise—it is the material left untouched by meaning.

Recognition Reversal: The recursive psychic phenomenon in which the very act of recognizing a psychic truth precipitates its alteration, dissociation, or symbolic undoing. Unlike repression, which hides before awareness, *Recognition Reversal* occurs *because* of awareness. To name is to shift structure. Insight brings truth *and* loss.

Recursive Mourning: A process in which the same loss is grieved repeatedly, each time with altered symbolic texture. Recursive Mourning honors that some losses are not linear—what was never fully had cannot be fully let go. Rather than closure, recursive mourning enacts symbolic rhythm: a circling that includes recognition, reversal, resistance, and return.

Subject as Symbol: The self is never simply a unified subject but a symbol of itself: condensed, refracted, partial, and offered. In this view, subjectivity is not a stable interior but a relational formation marked by absence and substitution. To live as a subject is to live as a stand-in—for what was lost, for what cannot be spoken, for what others need us to be.

Symbolic Intensity: Not affect alone, but affect rendered symbolically dense. Symbolic intensity describes moments when a word, a gesture, or a silence is saturated with multiple layers of meaning—not all of them knowable. It differs from emotional overwhelm: here, the intensity is structured, curated, and often ritualistic.

Symbolic Life: The dimension of psychic life that exceeds coherence. Symbolic life is not reducible to insight, narrative, or adaptation—it includes mystery, rupture, and aesthetic truth. It is what remains alive in the psyche even when structure fails. In analytic work, symbolic life is encountered through metaphor, silence, humor, eroticism, and dream.

Symbolic Saturation: A state in which the symbolic has become too full—where meaning presses so densely that affect collapses. It is not fragmentation, but its opposite: a symbolic field that allows no slippage. Often mistaken for insight, symbolic saturation suffocates the psychic breath. The task is to loosen—not interpret—the excess.

The Unformulated Third: A shared psychic field that exists between patient and analyst, but has not yet crystallized into language or concept. It is not the intersubjective "third" of mutual recognition, but a more fragile terrain: pre-symbolic, affective, and hovering. It is not unconscious content to be interpreted, but a field of possibility that precedes understanding.

Third Arc: The symbolic emergence that arises not from synthesis, but from recursive return. Where dialectics move toward resolution, the Third Arc moves in spirals. It is what emerges when paradox is *held*, not solved—when the analyst does not collapse ambiguity into coherence. It may appear as silence, aesthetic form, or the subtle realignment of subjectivity.

Undoing Fold: A topological image for the twist that occurs at the moment of psychic symbolization. Recognition and its undoing are not linear but folded into one another—each curve of knowing marked by a seam of destabilization. The Undoing Fold honors recursive disassembly. To speak is to fold.

Wise Baby: A prematurely observing ego formed not through development but through rupture. The Wise Baby is not a metaphor for giftedness but a dissociative formation—an internalized stance that sees too much, too soon, without containment. It witnesses an unbearable experience from a symbolic remove. The Wise Baby holds knowledge that the body hasn't yet survived.

Postscript—Recognition Reversal and the Architecture of Undoing

This postscript further explores *Recognition Reversal*, as initially discussed at the beginning of this book, as a fundamental yet overlooked structure of subjectivity, in which the act of becoming known coincides with symbolic undoing. Drawing from clinical process, myth, metapsychology, literature, and art, this chapter reframes the moment of recognition not as resolution, but as a recursive event in which psychic presence and self-cancellation co-arise. Recognition Reversal is proposed not as resistance or defense, but as a structural principle of symbolic life: to name is to estrange and to witness is to risk vanishing. By tracing this phenomenon across clinical vignettes, religious motifs, aesthetic practice, and philosophical recursion, this chapter positions reversal as an architectural necessity in the formation of subjectivity and a key to understanding the fragile, luminous edge of therapeutic contact.

Revisiting the Fold

Marcus had been speaking of his father—a man who vanished often without explanation, who returned with stories that never quite added up. There was no accusation in Marcus's tone, only a smooth indifference, the kind that sounds healed but smells of abandonment. We had circled this terrain for weeks, naming the loss but never touching it. Then, one afternoon, something flickered. He looked at me with a softness that startled us both and said: "I think I've always been waiting for someone to ask how it felt."

There was no silence after that line. There was quiet, yes—but not the kind that opens. The room felt still in a way that was not peaceful, but sealed. His affect dimmed. My breath slowed. Something in the field pulled away. In that moment—just when recognition had arrived—the recognition was gone.

This postscript begins where many analytic hours end: at the point of vanishing. The patient comes close to something, almost says it, or does say it, and then—retreats. Or the analyst finds the phrase that finally names the mood, only to discover the mood has fled. We are taught to call this resistance, defense, or dissociation. But what if something else is at work? What if the psyche does not simply *avoid* knowing, but is altered the moment it knows?

This chapter continues the exploration of a structure I introduced at the beginning of this book, called ***Recognition Reversal***: the co-arising of symbolization and undoing. It is not that insight kills the truth or that language fails the real. Rather, it is that the moment a psychic experience becomes recognizable, something essential about its *unknowingness*—its rawness, its immediacy, its charge—is reversed, recoiled, partially sealed. The recognition gives access; the reversal withdraws what was just glimpsed.

It is a structure, not a mistake.

Like the moment a dream is told and no longer feels alive.

Like the way a patient says, "that's exactly it," and then looks away.

Like the analyst who finds the perfect interpretation—only to feel something vital has just slipped from the field.

This is not failure. It is **architecture**. A recursive fold in the symbolic life of the mind. A gesture that marks not repression but subjectivity itself.

Recognition Reversal will not be proven in what follows. It has already happened. It happened in the chapters you've read—when the Wise Baby vanished into intellect, when erotic submission shimmered and then flattened, when aliveness flickered in a phrase and then curled into coherence. You may have felt it without naming it: a mood that passed through you, then unspooled, like a thread you could no longer find.

We begin this final chapter not to explain, but to return. To feel again that something in recognition always includes its own undoing—and that undoing, when held symbolically, may reveal the subject as it truly is: not coherent, but recursive; not whole, but held.

Defining Recognition Reversal

Recognition Reversal refers to the recursive psychic event in which the act of becoming known coincides with a partial dissolution of what is known. It is not a defense against insight, but a structural fold within symbolization itself. In this reversal, meaning does not retreat entirely—it is not undone like a lie exposed—but it shifts, warps, loses its immediacy. The affective charge drains. The object of recognition, having been named, becomes unreachable in its original form.

This is not repression, which operates by keeping certain contents unconscious. Nor is it resistance, which implies intentional or unconscious opposition to change. It is not even dissociation, though it shares its suddenness. Rather, *Recognition Reversal* describes a *co-arising event*: a moment in which psychic presence and symbolic withdrawal happen simultaneously. It is the psyche's paradoxical relationship to knowing: the truth must be found, and once found, it can no longer be held in the same way.

To recognize is to change the thing recognized.

To name is to estrange.

The reversal is not an error. It is what allows psychic life to remain symbolically alive. Without it, recognition would collapse into certainty; language would flatten affect; truth would become deadened fact. The reversal preserves movement. It keeps the subject from being fixed—even in the moment of being seen. The concept arises clinically in subtle, affectively loaded ways:

- A patient articulates a long-circling truth and immediately becomes self-conscious, ironic, or detached.
- A vivid dream is shared, only to be followed by days of silence or forgetfulness.
- The analyst's well-placed interpretation lands—then chills the room.

These are not simply moments of fragility or shame. They mark the activation of a deeper logic: that subjectivity is never stable under the gaze of recognition. The moment one is seen, one begins to withdraw. The moment something is known, it becomes something else. The reversal is not regression—it is transformation via recursive contact with symbolization itself.

This phenomenon is mirrored in literature and mysticism as well:

- In the Zen koan, where the insight flashes and then recedes.
- In Rilke's *Duino Elegies*, where the angel's unbearable clarity requires us to live among the partial and the dying.
- In mystical apophatic theology, where God is approached by what cannot be said, and every utterance reverses its own adequacy.

In psychoanalytic terms, *Recognition Reversal* can be read as a derivative of Laplanche's "message from the other" that carries an *enigmatic excess*—a message that, when translated, loses something essential in the very process of becoming comprehensible. It is also deeply aligned with Derrida's *différance*, where no sign ever fully arrives; every meaning is shadowed by what it displaces.

But here, the reversal is not just linguistic. It is clinical. Emotional. Symbolic. Lived.

Recognition Reversal is what occurs when the symbolic field flexes to accommodate meaning—and in doing so, pushes part of that meaning into shadow. It is the ripple that follows articulation, not because articulation failed, but because the psyche is structured to remain unstable in the face of knowing. The analyst must not rush to "keep the truth alive," as if recognition were a perishable fruit. The reversal *is* the aliveness.

To recognize is to touch. To reverse is to preserve the possibility of touching again.

Subjectivity as Self-Cancellation

What if the subject is not undone by accident, but by design?

What if to be a subject is already to be in partial flight from one's own recognition?

The idea that subjectivity is inherently divided is not new. Freud's unconscious, Lacan's barred subject, and Laplanche's enigmatic core—all point toward a psychic structure that cannot fully coincide with itself. But what Recognition Reversal adds to this tradition is a temporal and affective twist: that the moment of symbolic convergence—when something of the self becomes recognizable—is also the moment of dislocation. The self emerges not as presence, but as remainder.

The subject, in this view, is not only split but **self-cancelling**: it exists in and through symbolic operations that both sustain and undo it. This is not pathology. It is the very architecture of psychic life. To name the self is to mark the gap between being and being known.

Derrida gave us *différance*: the idea that every sign is marked by delay and difference, that meaning is always in motion, never fully present. Recognition Reversal can be read as its clinical cousin: not a theory of language alone, but a structure of **affective reversibility**, where psychic presence is always accompanied by its own eclipse.

Laplanche, too, gestures toward this with his theory of **the enigmatic signifier**: a message implanted by the adult unconscious into the child, saturated with meaning the child cannot yet decode. The child's translation—necessary for psychic survival—alters the message. The message that gives rise to subjectivity is also the one that **disfigures** it. Translation is the origin and the undoing.

From mathematics, Gödel's incompleteness theorem speaks to this in another register: no system can fully account for itself from within itself. There will always be a proposition that is true, but unprovable. The psyche, too, contains propositions—memories, affects, truths—that remain unformulated not because they are unknown, but because **they dissolve the moment they become knowable**. Gödel did not name the soul, but he mapped its architecture.

Even Loewald, who wrote so beautifully about the **internalization of the other** through symbolization, left room for this tension. He reminds us that the symbolized object is never the same as the object it replaces. There is always a gap—a transformation that carries both gain and loss. The psyche builds itself from these gaps. And every moment of internal coherence is haunted by the partiality it requires.

Subjectivity, then, is not a ground but a fold—a recursive curve formed by symbolic reversals. To say "I" is to reach for a coherence that reverses even as it arrives. This is not the self as illusion. It is the self as **oscillating surface**: flickering between contact and absence, symbol and remainder, presence and undoing.

We might say the subject is a wound dressed in language.

Or a name that forgets the body it once described.

Or a phrase that repeats itself, but never identically.

If this is true, then recognition—especially in the clinical encounter—can never be a simple gift. It is always a wound, a reach, and a disappearance.

It gives, it alters, and it leaves. What the analyst recognizes in the patient is not a fixed truth, but a contour that shimmers briefly before softening.

To witness *Recognition Reversal,* then, is not to stop it or resist it. It is to know that the self can only be known *as it begins to shift again*.

Myth and Ritual: Creation That Unmakes

Long before psychoanalysis attempted to name the fold in the psyche, myth had already lived in it.

Across cultures, the moment of creation is never pure. It arrives through rupture, violence, sacrifice, or contradiction. Subjectivity, in mythic form, is always born not just through emergence—but through **undoing**. In these stories, recognition does not stabilize the world—it fractures it. And the gods, like the analysand, are always trying to survive the aftermath of being seen.

Take **Dionysus**. He is not simply the god of wine and pleasure, but of ecstasy, madness, and dismemberment. In the Orphic tradition, the infant Dionysus is torn apart by the Titans and later reassembled from the surviving heart. The god who is whole is made of parts. He becomes divine not by avoiding fragmentation, but by *being shattered and returned to*. Recognition—his being seen by the Titans—leads to his death. But it is also the condition of his rebirth. The reversal is not the opposite of creation; it is its route.

Or consider **Shiva**, the Hindu god who dances the world into being and simultaneously destroys it. His movement is circular, recursive—each gesture a cycle of manifestation and dissolution. Shiva is worshiped as the *Nataraja*, Lord of the Dance, whose foot crushes ignorance even as his fire incinerates the cosmos. To witness him is to know that what is brought into form is already vanishing. He is recognition made visible—and therefore, already reversing.

In **Genesis**, Adam is given the task of naming the animals—a gesture often read as the birth of human consciousness and mastery over the world. But naming is also separation. Each word divides what was once whole. And the moment Adam names Eve, she is no longer simply flesh of his flesh—she is Other. Knowledge is estrangement. The Fall does not begin with the fruit—it begins with the utterance. With the symbol.

Even the **Ouroboros**, the serpent who eats its own tail, has long been a symbol of totality—but only through recursion. It does not stabilize. It devours. The cycle of self-consumption is what sustains its form. It lives by undoing itself.

These myths not only illustrate Recognition Reversal, but they *embody* it. In each, something is brought into being that cannot remain intact. To be seen, to be named, to be touched by symbolic presence—these are not events of completion. They are acts of tension, of rupture. They are what make us and what unmake us.

Rituals, too, follow this logic. The mourning ritual enacts a loss that is already felt but not yet spoken. The wedding ritual names a union that transforms the lovers from who they were. The baptismal plunge and the mikveh immersion both cleanse and erase. These are not acts of stabilization—they are **threshold enactments**. Each gesture marks that the self who enters will not be the self who leaves.

Analytic ritual is no different. The couch, the hour, the frame, the silence—they make possible a kind of symbolic becoming that undoes as it reveals. When a patient finally says what they have never said aloud, the ritual holds it—and yet, the affect may soften. The charge may go. What was alive becomes *form*. The reversal is not a failure of the setting. It is its mythic function.

Recognition Reversal, then, is not only a clinical phenomenon—it is a ritual one. A mythic one. A symbolic one. It marks the cost of entering the symbolic order: what is gained in articulation is always shadowed by what is lost in immediacy.

We do not recover the self by finding it. We recover it by **losing it in a new way**, again and again, across myth, ritual, and analysis.

And perhaps that is the real task of the analyst—not to preserve the truth, but to accompany the subject as they **pass through their own reversals**, trusting that something—if not preserved—will recur.

Literature, Art, and the Fragility of Form

Art has always known what theory forgets: that the moment a thing becomes visible, it begins to disappear. *Recognition Reversal* is not only a psychoanalytic or mythic structure—it is an aesthetic one. Literature, painting, music—all carry the trace of their own undoing. They show the thing, and in showing, alter it. They hold the subject in view just long enough for it to dissolve.

Take **Paul Celan**, whose poems bear the syntax of trauma—where language strains to say what has already been erased. In his late work, meaning hovers at the edge of formulation. A line lands like an incision, then reverses itself in silence. The reader recognizes something but cannot hold it. The poem recedes. This is not obfuscation. It is the form speaking its reversal.

Ingeborg Bachmann, too, wrote of language as both home and exile. Her words carve a subject who is always in motion, always slipping the frame. In her novel *Malina*, the narrator writes toward recognition—and ends with disappearance, with a final line that names her absence: *"It was murder."* The clarity arrives too late. Or perhaps, just in time to undo what was briefly found.

Rainer Maria Rilke, in the *Duino Elegies*, touches the unbearable beauty of what must die. His angels are not comforting—they are terrifying precisely because they see too much. The poem becomes a space where truth flares and falters. Rilke does not close the form—he lets it tremble.

Visual art, too, enacts this fold. In the late works of **Rothko**, the canvas becomes a field of absorption. The viewer stands before a depth that cannot be stabilized. The more one looks, the more the edges shift. Color becomes mood, then atmosphere, then nothing. The moment of recognition—*this is* *red, this is presence*—recedes into affective indeterminacy. Rothko's paintings are rituals of symbolic disappearance.

Agnes Martin, with her grids and muted tones, created paintings that seem to disappear as you approach them. She once said, "Beauty is the mystery of life. It is not in the eye—it is in the mind." Her work is an invitation to lose one's bearings—to recognize a structure that evaporates under contact. To be moved, and then to wonder if anything moved at all.

Music may be the most temporal form of reversal. In **Webern's** short, fragmented compositions, a motif emerges and is gone before it can be known. In **Beethoven's** late quartets, especially the *Cavatina* of Opus 130, the line stretches toward meaning and then falters, weeps, pauses. The beauty is unbearable, not because it fails, but because it *knows it cannot last*.

These works do not merely illustrate *Recognition Reversal*—they enact it. They stage the process by which form gives way to formlessness, and meaning flickers into unmaking. They are not expressions of despair, but of precision: to know that what can be touched must, in the same movement, slip away.

The artist, like the analyst, is not seeking to preserve. They are seeking to **stay with**—to hold the shimmer before it breaks, to track the edge of form as it folds. Not to fix what is vanishing, but to witness the reversal as structure, not loss.

Recognition Reversal, then, belongs to aesthetics as much as to analysis. To read, to paint, to compose, to dream—these are all acts of symbolic contact and retreat. The beauty lies not in the holding, but in the **receding curve**—where meaning leaves just enough residue to make the next return possible.

Clinical Reversals: Knowing That Vanishes

In the analytic room, *Recognition Reversal* is not a concept. It is an atmosphere. A subtle shift. A sudden thinning of presence, a dimming of heat, a clarity that gives way to detachment.

It is the moment the truth arrives—and then leaves.

Marcus, again. After naming his grief—finally, carefully—his tone went faintly cheerful. "It's funny, really. I always thought I was fine." The pain we had spent months approaching was suddenly bracketed, wrapped, and returned to narrative. But something in the room had changed. The earlier tension had evaporated. He had not repressed the truth—he had *survived it symbolically*, and in doing so, could no longer touch it.

Or Eden, who had described the erotic thrill of surrendering to a partner's will: "It's like disappearing into someone else's desire—I don't have to be a self anymore." Her voice rang with clarity, almost glee. But in the next session, she was blank and irritable. "I don't know what we're doing here," she said. The moment of contact had curdled. The truth had reversed.

Or Jonas, whose accommodating choreography had finally slipped. He noticed himself caretaking a friend and said, in session, "I do this with everyone. It's like I disappear unless I'm helping." His eyes watered. Then he laughed, sarcastic: "How original. Textbook." And the moment was gone.

These are not failures of interpretation, nor regressions in development. They are **reversals of recognition**, embedded in the structure of symbolization itself. The affect, once spoken, loses intensity. The insight, once named, becomes clinical knowledge—organized, lifeless. The analyst, if too eager, might miss the reversal and try to resuscitate the earlier feeling. But the reversal cannot be undone. It is not a retreat from contact—it *is* contact, inverted.

What matters is not preventing the reversal, but **staying with its arc**.

Some patients reverse subtly: a glaze in the eye, a change in posture. Others shift dramatically: anger, shutdown, disengagement. These shifts are often read diagnostically—as resistance, splitting, narcissistic injury. But they can also be read **structurally**, as part of the psyche's way of metabolizing symbolic contact. The reversal is not avoidance—it is the psyche's way of surviving knowing.

For the analyst, the task is not to push against the reversal, nor to rush toward re-integration. It is to **recognize the reversal as meaningful in itself**.

To say:

I feel you pulling back after coming close. Let's stay near that edge.

Or even simply: Something shifted—can we feel that together?

When spoken gently, without intrusion, this acknowledgment does not stop the reversal—but it allows it to be witnessed. The reversal becomes not a disappearance, but a **shared symbolic fold**. What had been solitary—unknowable—is now *reversibly known*, not as content, but as form.

Recognition Reversal, in the clinic, reminds us that insight is not a destination. It is a passage. A clearing. And often, a veiling.

It asks us to listen for what slips—not just what is said.

To witness what vanishes—not just what arrives.

To trust that the reversal is not an erasure of contact, but its deepening.

Sometimes the most honest thing the analyst can do is sit in the stillness that follows a recognition and say nothing—knowing that what just came into view is already folding itself away, and that this, too, is the work.

A Remained Gesture

Recognition Reversal is not the final concept of this book. It is what remains when the others have unfolded.

It lingers like the aftertaste of an interpretation too true to repeat. It hovers behind the clinical moment that felt whole—until the next hour, when its seams begin to show. It is what the patient forgets after remembering and what the analyst senses as a shift without words. It is the reversal not of truth, but of symbolized presence—the unmaking that holds the possibility of meaning.

I have not tried to systematize it. You've already read its shape in earlier chapters—in the loops and fragments, in the soft recursions, in the silences between resolution and remainder. This chapter does not explain the book; it enacts what the book has always known: that each act of symbolic contact bears within it the trace of its own reversal.

To name something is to estrange it.

To touch a truth is to feel it begin to dissolve.

To be witnessed is to disappear, slightly, into the act of being seen.

This is not a flaw. It is the design.

The architecture of subjectivity is recursive, unstable, luminous. It folds back on itself to preserve what cannot yet be known in full. Recognition Reversal is not a mistake of the analytic process—it is its pulse. It is how the psyche keeps moving, even after the words arrive.

There is no conclusion to this book. No final integration.

Instead, let it end as it began—in a mood, a tension, a fold.

Perhaps, even now, something you thought you understood in an earlier chapter has begun to blur. Let it. That soft undoing is not confusion. It is the symbolic structure reasserting its life. What vanishes may still return, in another form, another hour, another sentence.

So let this be not an ending, but a **remained gesture**—a phrase that slips as it lands.

What you recognize here may already be gone.

But what was reversed may someday recur and shimmer again.

Bibliography

Agamben, G. (1998). *Homo sacer: Sovereign power and bare life* (D. Heller-Roazen, Trans.). Stanford University Press.

Akhtar, S. (1998). From simplicity through contradiction to paradox: The evolving psychic reality of the borderline patient in treatment. *The International Journal of Psychoanalysis, 79*(2), 241–252.

Atlas, G. (2022). *Emotional inheritance: A therapist, her patients, and the legacy of trauma*. Little, Brown Spark.

Bachmann, I. (1990). *Malina* (P. Boehm, Trans.). Holmes & Meier.

Barad, K. (2007). *Meeting the universe halfway: Quantum physics and the entanglement of matter and meaning*. Duke University Press.

Beebe, B., Lachmann, F., & Jaffe, J. (1997). Mother–infant interaction structures and presymbolic self- and object representations. *Psychoanalytic Dialogues, 7*(2), 133–182.

Benjamin, J. (1988). *The bonds of love: Psychoanalysis, feminism, and the problem of domination*. Pantheon Books.

Benjamin, J. (1990). An outline of intersubjectivity: The development of recognition. *Psychoanalytic Psychology, 7*(Suppl.), 33–46.

Benjamin, J. (1995). *Like subjects, love objects: Essays on recognition and sexual difference*. Yale University Press.

Benjamin, J. (1998). *Shadow of the other: Intersubjectivity and gender in psychoanalysis*. Routledge.

Benjamin, J. (2004). Beyond doer and done to: An intersubjective view of thirdness. *The Psychoanalytic Quarterly, 73*(1), 5–46.

Bion, W. R. (1962). *Learning from experience*. Heinemann.

Bollas, C. (1987). *The shadow of the object: Psychoanalysis of the unthought known*. Columbia University Press.

Bollas, C. (1992). *Being a character: Psychoanalysis and self experience*. Hill & Wang.

Brandchaft, B., Stolorow, R. D., & Atwood, G. E. (2010). *Structures of subjectivity: Explorations in psychoanalytic phenomenology and contextualism* (2nd ed.). Routledge. (Original work published 1994).

Bromberg, P. M. (1998). *Standing in the spaces: Essays on clinical process, trauma, and dissociation*. Analytic Press.

Bromberg, P. M. (2006). *Awakening the dreamer: Clinical journeys*. Analytic Press.

Buber, M. (1970). *I and Thou* (W. Kaufmann, Trans.). Charles Scribner's Sons. (Original work published 1923).

Butler, J. (2005). *Giving an account of oneself*. Fordham University Press.
Celan, P. (2001). *Selected poems and prose of Paul Celan* (J. Felstiner, Trans.). W. W. Norton.
Chasseguet-Smirgel, J. (1985). *Creativity and perversion*. Free Association Books.
Damasio, A. R. (1994). *Descartes' error: Emotion, reason, and the human brain*. G. P. Putnam's Sons.
Damasio, A. R. (1999). *The feeling of what happens: Body and emotion in the making of consciousness*. Harcourt.
Dean, T. (2000). *Beyond sexuality*. University of Chicago Press.
Derrida, J. (1976). *Of grammatology* (G. C. Spivak, Trans.). Johns Hopkins University Press. (Original work published 1967).
Derrida, J. (1978). *Writing and difference* (A. Bass, Trans.). University of Chicago Press. (Original work published 1967).
Derrida, J. (1995). *The gift of death* (D. Wills, Trans.). University of Chicago Press.
Dimen, M. (2003). *Sexuality, intimacy, power*. Analytic Press.
Eigen, M. (1986). *The psychotic core*. Jason Aronson.
Eigen, M. (1998). *The psychoanalytic mystic*. Free Association Books.
Eigen, M. (2004). *The sensitive self*. Wesleyan University Press.
Eigen, M. (2011). *Contact with the depths*. Routledge.
Epstein, M. (1995). *Thoughts without a thinker: Psychotherapy from a Buddhist perspective*. Basic Books.
Ettinger, B. L. (2006). *The matrixial borderspace*. University of Minnesota Press.
Fairbairn, W. R. D. (1943). The repression and the return of bad objects (with special reference to the 'war neuroses'). In D. E. Scharff (Ed.), *Foundations of object relations theory* (pp. 65–89). Jason Aronson.
Fairbairn, W. R. D. (1944). Endopsychic structure considered in terms of object relationships. *International Journal of Psychoanalysis*, *25*, 70–92.
Fairbairn, W. R. D. (1952). *Psychoanalytic studies of the personality*. Routledge.
Fanon, F. (1967). *Black skin, white masks* (C. L. Markmann, Trans.). Grove Press. (Original work published 1952).
Ferenczi, S. (1933). Confusion of tongues between the adults and the child. *International Journal of Psychoanalysis*, *30*, 225–230.
Fonagy, P., Luyten, P., & Allison, E. (2015). Epistemic petrification and the restoration of epistemic trust: A new conceptualization of borderline personality disorder and its treatment. *Journal of Personality Disorders*, *29*(5), 575–609.
Foucault, M. (1977). *Discipline and punish: The birth of the prison* (A. Sheridan, Trans.). Pantheon Books.
Foucault, M. (1978). *The history of sexuality, Vol. 1: An introduction* (R. Hurley, Trans.). Pantheon Books.
Freud, S. (1953a). Fragment of an analysis of a case of hysteria. In J. Strachey (Ed. & Trans.), *The standard edition of the complete psychological works of Sigmund Freud* (Vol. 7, pp. 1–122). Hogarth Press. (Original work published 1905).
Freud, S. (1953b). Three essays on the theory of sexuality. In J. Strachey (Ed. & Trans.), *The standard edition of the complete psychological works of Sigmund Freud* (Vol. 7, pp. 123–246). Hogarth Press. (Original work published 1905).
Freud, S. (1955a). Analysis of a phobia in a five-year-old boy. In J. Strachey (Ed. & Trans.), *The standard edition of the complete psychological works of Sigmund Freud* (Vol. 10, pp. 1–149). Hogarth Press. (Original work published 1909).

Freud, S. (1955b). Beyond the pleasure principle. In J. Strachey (Ed. & Trans.), *The standard edition of the complete psychological works of Sigmund Freud* (Vol. 18, pp. 1–64). Hogarth Press. (Original work published 1920).
Freud, S. (1957a). On the universal tendency to debasement in the sphere of love. In J. Strachey (Ed. & Trans.), *The standard edition of the complete psychological works of Sigmund Freud* (Vol. 11, pp. 177–190). Hogarth Press. (Original work published 1912).
Freud, S. (1957b). The unconscious. In J. Strachey (Ed. & Trans.), *The standard edition of the complete psychological works of Sigmund Freud* (Vol. 14, pp. 159–215). Hogarth Press. (Original work published 1915).
Freud, S. (1961). The economic problem of masochism. In J. Strachey (Ed. & Trans.), *The standard edition of the complete psychological works of Sigmund Freud* (Vol. 19, pp. 155–172). Hogarth Press. (Original work published 1924).
Gödel, K. (1931). Über formal unentscheidbare Sätze der Principia Mathematica und verwandter Systeme I. *Monatshefte für Mathematik und Physik, 38*(1), 173–198.
Guntrip, H. (1961). *Personality structure and human interaction*. Hogarth Press.
Guntrip, H. (1969). *Schizoid phenomena, object relations and the self*. International Universities Press.
Harris, A. (2005). Gender as soft assembly. *Studies in Gender and Sexuality, 6*(1), 87–105.
Harris, A. (2009). The logic of therapeutic action in a time of crisis. *Psychoanalytic Dialogues, 19*(5), 620–637.
Heidegger, M. (1962). *Being and time* (J. Macquarrie & E. Robinson, Trans.). Harper & Row. (Original work published 1927).
Hoffman, I. Z. (1998). *Ritual and spontaneity in the psychoanalytic process: A dialectical-constructivist view*. Routledge.
Hofstadter, D. R. (1979). *Gödel, Escher, Bach: An eternal golden braid*. Basic Books.
Kernberg, O. F. (1975). *Borderline conditions and pathological narcissism*. Jason Aronson.
Kernberg, O. F. (1984). *Severe personality disorders: Psychotherapeutic strategies*. Yale University Press.
Khan, M. M. R. (1974). *The privacy of the self: Papers of psychoanalytic theory and technique*. Hogarth Press.
Khan, M. M. R. (1983). *Hidden selves: Between theory and practice in psychoanalysis*. International Universities Press.
Klein, M. (1946). Notes on some schizoid mechanisms. *The International Journal of Psycho-Analysis, 27*(3–4), 99–110.
Klein, M. (1975). *Envy and gratitude and other works 1946–1963* (Vol. 3). Hogarth Press.
Kristeva, J. (1982). *Powers of horror: An essay on abjection* (L. S. Roudiez, Trans.). Columbia University Press.
Kuchuck, S. (2021). The supervisor's body: Countertransference, enactment, and ethical intimacy. *Journal of the American Psychoanalytic Association, 69*(6), 1033–1051.
Laing, R. D. (1960). *The divided self: An existential study in sanity and madness*. Tavistock Publications.
Laing, R. D. (1961). *Self and others*. Tavistock Publications.
Laplanche, J. (1999). *Essays on otherness* (J. Fletcher, Trans.). Routledge.
Levinas, E. (1969). *Totality and infinity: An essay on exteriority* (A. Lingis, Trans.). Duquesne University Press. (Original work published 1961).

Loewald, H. W. (1978a). *Psychoanalysis and the history of the individual*. Yale University Press.
Loewald, H. W. (1978b). Psychoanalysis as a developmental process. In *Psychoanalysis and the history of the individual* (pp. 102–123). Yale University Press.
Loewald, H. W. (1978c). Internalization, separation, mourning, and the superego. In *Psychoanalysis and the history of the individual* (pp. 150–184). Yale University Press.
Loewald, H. W. (1978d). Primary process, secondary process, and reality. In *Psychoanalysis and the history of the individual* (pp. 111–127). Yale University Press.
Lorenzer, A. (1981). *Sprachzerstörung und Rekonstruktion: Vorarbeiten zu einer Metatheorie der Psychoanalyse*. Suhrkamp.
Mahler, M. S., Pine, F., & Bergman, A. (1975). *The psychological birth of the human infant: Symbiosis and individuation*. Basic Books.
McWilliams, N. (2011). *Psychoanalytic diagnosis: Understanding personality structure in the clinical process* (2nd ed.). Guilford Press.
Merleau-Ponty, M. (1962). *Phenomenology of perception* (C. Smith, Trans.). Routledge & Kegan Paul.
Mitchell, S. A. (1988). *Relational concepts in psychoanalysis: An integration*. Harvard University Press.
Mitchell, S. A. (1993). *Hope and dread in psychoanalysis*. Basic Books.
Mitchell, S. A. (2004). *Influence and autonomy in psychoanalysis*. Routledge. (Original work published 1997, Analytic Press).
Muñoz, J. E. (2009). *Cruising utopia: The then and there of queer futurity*. NYU Press.
Ogden, T. H. (1994). The analytic third: Working with intersubjective clinical facts. *The International Journal of Psycho-Analysis*, *75*(1), 3–19.
Ogden, T. H. (1997). Reverie and interpretation. *The Psychoanalytic Quarterly*, *66*(4), 567–595.
Ogden, T. H. (2005a). On psychoanalytic supervision. *The International Journal of Psycho-Analysis*, *86*(5), 1265–1280.
Ogden, T. H. (2005b). On the undreamt dream. *The Psychoanalytic Quarterly*, *74*(1), 49–67.
Ogden, T. H. (2005c). On the countertransference. *International Journal of Psychoanalysis*, *86*(4), 857–873.
Ogden, T. H. (2019). Ontological psychoanalysis or "what do you want to be when you grow up?" *The Psychoanalytic Quarterly*, *88*(4), 661–684.
Ogden, T. H. (2021). *Coming to life in the consulting room*. Routledge.
Ogden, T. H. (2024a). Ontological psychoanalysis in clinical practice. *The Psychoanalytic Quarterly*, *93*(1), 13–31.
Ogden, T. H. (2024b). *What alive means*. Routledge.
Orange, D. M. (1995). *Emotional understanding: Studies in psychoanalytic epistemology*. Guilford Press.
Orange, D. M. (2010). *Thinking for clinicians: Philosophical resources for contemporary psychoanalysis and the humanistic psychotherapies*. Routledge.
Panksepp, J. (1998). *Affective neuroscience: The foundations of human and animal emotions*. Oxford University Press.
Pellegrini, A. (2007). *Performance anxieties: Staging psychoanalysis, staging race*. Routledge.
Phillips, A. (1994). *On flirtation: Psychoanalytic essays on the unseen and unspoken*. Harvard University Press.
Phillips, A. (1996). *Terrors and experts*. Harvard University Press.

Phillips, A. (1998). *The beast in the nursery: On curiosity and other appetites*. Vintage.
Rank, O. (1929). *The trauma of birth*. Brace. (Original work published 1924).
Rank, O. (1936). *Will therapy, truth, and reality*. Knopf.
Reich, W. (1949). *Character analysis* (3rd ed., T. P. Wolfe, Trans.). Farrar, Straus & Giroux. (Original work published 1933).
Rilke, R. M. (2009). *Duino elegies* (E. Snow, Trans.). North Point Press.
Sedgwick, E. K. (1990). *Epistemology of the closet*. University of California Press.
Sedgwick, E. K. (2003). *Touching feeling: Affect, pedagogy, performativity*. Duke University Press.
Shapiro, R. (2020). Presence and dissociation: Working with patients who cannot tell the story. *Journal of the American Psychoanalytic Association*, *68*(1), 67–92.
Solms, M., & Turnbull, O. (2002). *The brain and the inner world: An introduction to the neuroscience of subjective experience*. Other Press.
Stern, D. B. (1997). *Unformulated experience: From dissociation to imagination in psychoanalysis*. Analytic Press.
Stern, D. B. (2003). *Unformulated experience: From dissociation to imagination in psychoanalysis*. Routledge. (Original work published 1997).
Stern, D. B. (2015). *Relational freedom: Emergent properties of the interpersonal field*. Routledge.
Stern, D. B. (2018). *The infinity of the unsaid: Unformulated experience, language, and the nonverbal*. Routledge.
Stern, D. N. (1985). *The interpersonal world of the infant: A view from psychoanalysis and developmental psychology*. Basic Books.
Stern, D. N. (2010). *Forms of vitality: Exploring dynamic experience in psychology, the arts, psychotherapy, and development*. Oxford University Press.
Stolorow, R. D. (2007). *Trauma and human existence: Autobiographical, psychoanalytic, and philosophical reflections*. Routledge.
Stolorow, R. D., Atwood, G. E., & Brandchaft, B. (2002). *Worlds of experience: Interweaving philosophical and clinical dimensions in psychoanalysis*. Basic Books.
Stolorow, R. D., & Brandchaft, B. (2010). *The intersubjective perspective*. Jason Aronson.
Stolorow, R. D., Brandchaft, B., & Atwood, G. E. (1987). *Psychoanalytic treatment: An intersubjective approach*. Analytic Press.
Sullivan, H. S. (1953). *The interpersonal theory of psychiatry*. W. W. Norton.
Winnicott, D. W. (1953). Transitional objects and transitional phenomena. *International Journal of Psycho-Analysis*, *34*, 89–97.
Winnicott, D. W. (1965). *The maturational processes and the facilitating environment: Studies in the theory of emotional development*. International Universities Press.
Winnicott, D. W. (1974). Fear of breakdown. *International Review of Psychoanalysis*, *1*, 103–107.
Winnicott, D. W. (1986). *Home is where we start from: Essays by D. W. Winnicott*. W. W. Norton.
Wittgenstein, L. (1953). *Philosophical investigations* (G. E. M. Anscombe, Trans.). Basil Blackwell.
Wittgenstein, L. (2001). *Tractatus logico-philosophicus* (D. F. Pears & B. F. McGuinness, Trans.). Routledge. (Original work published 1922).
Wynter, S. (2003). Unsettling the coloniality of being/power/truth/freedom: Towards the human, after man, its overrepresentation—An argument. *CR: The New Centennial Review*, *3*(3), 257–337.

Index

For Product Safety Concerns and Information please contact our EU
representative GPSR@taylorandfrancis.com
Taylor & Francis Verlag GmbH, Kaufingerstraße 24, 80331 München, Germany

www.ingramcontent.com/pod-product-compliance
Ingram Content Group UK Ltd.
Pitfield, Milton Keynes, MK11 3LW, UK
UKHW020009200926
475702UK00015B/2564
* 9 7 8 1 0 4 1 1 7 1 4 8 5 *